STRENGTH TRAINING
OVER 40

STRENGTH TRAINING OVER 40

A 6-Week Program to Build Muscle and Agility

ALANA COLLINS

Illustration by Mat Edwards

ROCKRIDGE PRESS

Interior and Cover Designer: Jami Spittler   Editor: Rochelle Torke and Nicky Montalvo

Art Producer: Karen Williams   Production Editor: Ruth Sakata Corley

Illustration © 2020 Mat Edwards

ISBN: Print 978-1-64611-612-6 | eBook 978-1-64611-613-3

R1

This is for Joshua and Benjamin.
They are my "why."

INTRODUCTION

I have been a certified strength training coach since 2012, working primarily with women and men over the age of 40, and have been in the gym most of my adult life. At 62, I can honestly say that I'm in the best shape of my life, and I attribute that almost exclusively to strength training. You've chosen this book, which means that maintaining a strong body is important to you, too. It's my hope that this book will be a simple yet thorough guide for your commitment to building and maintaining strength in your body, which will in turn enable you to do all of those things you love to do for years to come. I congratulate you for being open-minded enough to give this form of exercise a chance.

Middle-age weight gain is directly tied to our loss of muscle mass, which begins for most of us in our mid-thirties. If we maintain our muscle mass, we keep our metabolism revved up. It's a win-win!

As you age, you may notice joint pain and weight gain setting in. Perhaps your range of motion isn't what it used to be. You may have been told that your bone density isn't what it ought to be. Maybe it's more difficult maintaining good posture or that simple tasks take more energy, if you're able to do them at all. Or you've noticed a general weakness and tiring of the body or lax skin where muscle once was and accept it as an inevitable part of aging. But that doesn't have to be the case. The most heartening thing about strength training is that our bodies *want* to be strong. All we need to do is provide the stimulus.

HOW TO USE THIS BOOK

By the end of this book, you will have completed six weeks of comprehensive strength training. I encourage you to start at the beginning and work through the book in the order in which it is written. The first chapters will help prepare you for a strong start and allow you to maintain your fitness after the six weeks is concluded.

You will find workout programs and tutorials for each exercise so that you can be sure that you're getting the most out of each exercise in a way that won't put your body at risk for injury.

We'll focus on well-balanced, full-body workouts that you can do in the gym or at home beginning with a manageable 30-minute time frame; however, workouts can be adjusted, depending on your current fitness level.

Along with the exercise name, you will be given the muscles that are being targeted. If you're like me, you'll be more motivated to do the exercise if you're aware of the benefits of that movement. You'll have step-by-step instructions along with a less challenging alternative, if that's what you need.

You'll also be given a safety tip and general pointers for the exercise when necessary, because keeping you safe and injury-free is my goal. Illustrations that demonstrate the exercises, combined with the tutorial page number, will make this process super easy for you!

Starting Strong

LIVE LONG AND STRONG

We are told that we need to strengthen our bodies, but it isn't always clear to us why muscle strength is so important. In this chapter I will break down the reasons why we need to maintain, and in many cases rebuild, our muscle mass.

Perhaps you thought that those people who go to the gym were there purely for vanity reasons. That couldn't be further from the truth. There are numerous reasons strength training is imperative for our health, and it's time we had a better understanding of just why that is.

TIME, YOUR BODY, AND THE SECRET WEAPON

Physically inactive people will begin to lose a small percentage of muscle each decade after their 30s, which contributes to general weakness and lower quality of life. This is a natural process known as sarcopenia.

Many people believe that activities such as walking, cycling, or swimming will be enough to keep their muscles strong. But this is not the case. While these activities are certainly beneficial, they are not enough to keep your muscle mass intact.

Adding resistance training will retain your strength, improve your appearance, balance, and posture, and enable you to continue doing the activities you enjoy.

We must place a new demand on our muscles so they get the signal that you require more from them. I love the expression "Change doesn't happen in your comfort zone," and this is true for building muscle just as it is for our personal growth.

After you work out with added resistance, your body repairs and replaces damaged muscle fibers; but the great thing is, this muscle builds back *stronger* than it was in order to accommodate the new demands. Change doesn't happen overnight, but it *will* happen. As I often tell my clients, your body can't help but get stronger if you continue to place those demands on it in a safe and consistent manner.

Muscle knows no age, but the sooner you start, the better quality of life you'll have in your 40s, 50s, 60s, and well beyond!

THE MUSCLE, HORMONE, AND METABOLISM CONNECTION

Strength training triggers the production of the hormones that control our metabolism as well as help us develop muscle. We're learning that our musculoskeletal system serves as a sort of endocrine organ that plays a key role in metabolism.

In recent years, the hormones insulin and cortisol have become part of the conversation about body composition. We've begun to realize that getting lean is not as simple as "calories in versus calories out." When it comes to changing your fat-to-muscle ratio, both calories and hormones matter, particularly as we age. While we need to be in a caloric deficit (taking in fewer calories than we're burning) for your stored energy to be used as fuel, managing cravings when we're trying to cut calories has more to do with hormones.

The fact that strength training can drive insulin levels down means that levels can normalize while cortisol is kept in check. Being that there seems to be a connection between cortisol and estrogen dominance (which can worsen for many women as we approach menopause), it's important to keep both insulin and cortisol in normal ranges. When cortisol is elevated for extended periods of time, it can cause negative health issues, including increased belly fat.

Older people tend to be more insulin-resistant, but there is controversy regarding the reasons for this. Is it an inevitable part of aging or the result of lifestyle choices? Personally, I would bet that insulin resistance has more to do with lifestyle choices and is responsible for increased risk of type 2 diabetes as well as heart attacks, strokes, and cancer.

The bottom line is that strength training is the most powerful tool for building muscle and losing fat. There are no alternatives and no shortcuts. By recompositioning our body in this way, we will be better able to manage our hormone levels and keep that complicated endocrine system in excellent order as we age. Additionally, there is the fundamental fact that muscle burns more calories than fat. This means that the more muscle tissue you have, the more calories your body burns, even at rest.

BONE DENSITY

Most people know that strength training, whether with body weight, dumbbells, barbells, kettlebells, or resistance bands, can build muscle and strength. But did you know that by strengthening our muscles we also strengthen our bones, which in turn helps minimize osteoporosis? Osteoporosis is the loss of calcium and other minerals from a person's bones, which makes the bones susceptible to fracturing.

A sedentary lifestyle is the biggest contributor to the loss of bone mass as we age. Bone loss is estimated at a rate of approximately one percent per year after about the age of 40, *if* we don't purposefully work against it. The more significant the loss of bone density, the more susceptible we are to fracturing a bone, even while doing a simple task.

The great news is strength training can seriously slow bone loss, and as some studies have shown, can even rebuild bone. When first consulting with a new client who has been diagnosed with osteopenia or osteoporosis, I'm always happy to learn that their physician recommended strength training, rather than putting them on medication or simply recommending a calcium supplement.

A "weight-bearing exercise" is a form of exercise that will help offset osteoporosis. Weight-bearing activity places stress on bones by creating a tugging action, which in turn can stimulate the growth of bone cells. The best way to create this tugging action is through strength training, although you'll gain some benefits with aerobic activities such as walking, hiking, jogging, playing racquet sports, and even dancing. However, if you have a serious concern regarding bone loss, strength training has the greatest regenerative effect, by targeting bones in a purposeful way.

One of the most heartwarming parts of my job is witnessing my clients gain the wonderful sense of confidence that comes with gaining a stronger, more stable body. This confidence seems to propel them into new activities and serves to fulfill social and emotional aspects of their lives as well as their physical fitness.

STRENGTH, BALANCE, AND MOBILITY

Strength, along with balance, affects our ability to move in a functional manner; therefore, if our mobility is limited, due to decreased balance and strength, we will be at risk for the general deterioration of our structural bodies, as well as the emotional components that will likely accompany the loss of function.

If we allow our muscles to atrophy to the point of noticeable muscle loss and weakness, then both balance and mobility *will* be affected.

Good balance requires the coordination of several parts of the body, including muscles, bones, and joints. There are also other issues that can affect balance, such as poor eyesight or inner ear problems, but if we maintain our strength and range of motion, we will be less apt to lose our balance in the first place, and better able to recover if we do. Balance as we age is crucial. One of the leading causes of injury to aged individuals is falls.

The combination of strength, balance, and mobility equals stability, and stability equals a strong and sturdy body. Strengthening movements with free weights require stability so that your stabilizing muscles must kick in to help, and they in turn get stronger, along with the targeted muscle group. For example, by doing exercises one leg at a time, you're required to balance if even for only a second or two, which requires the use of our hip stabilizers. By incorporating the hip stabilizers, we not only strengthen the muscles surrounding the hip joints, but we help create a more stable body in general.

These days there isn't as much emphasis on flexibility as there once was. Instead, we focus on maintaining our *natural range* of motion in combination with strength. While it is important to maintain our natural range of motion, to stretch *beyond* that point can do more harm than good. An increase in flexibility without strength results in joint instability. So once again we see the importance of keeping our muscles strong.

BRAIN HEALTH

In recent years, various studies have shown that greater muscle strength is associated with better cognitive function in aging men and women. Cognition refers to brain functions relating to receiving, storing, processing, and using information. These findings were published in the *European Geriatric Medicine Journal*.

Scientists at Florida Atlantic University found that sarcopenia and obesity (independently, but especially when occurring together) can heighten the risk of cognitive function impairments later in life. These results were published in the journal *Clinical Interventions in Aging*. Meanwhile, a 2012 University of British Columbia study published in the *Archives of Internal Medicine* compared cardio exercise and strength training in a randomized, controlled trial. Neuroimaging of the brain showed that the areas responsible for memory and executive function were more active after strength training.

This study showed that older adults who did both cardio *and* strength training were generally healthier compared to those who only did yoga and Pilates. But this study's most significant finding was that those people who did the *most* amount of weight training showed significantly fewer lesions in the brain. The study concluded that lifting weights is beneficial to overall brain health.

It's safe to say that strength training is good for us for so many reasons, including having neuroprotective properties. Lifting weights not only helps us regain physical strength and rev up our metabolism but it helps us retain a healthy brain as well!

chapter 2

YOU'VE GOT THIS!

It's important to take it upon ourselves to learn about fitness and nutrition, because knowledge really is power. Our bodies are amazing machines and the more we learn about how they function, the more apt we are to take good care of them.

Remember that there is no magic pill, potion, or product that will do the work for you. At the outset, there *will* be some trial and error as you embark upon your new lifestyle. When you make a mistake, or fall off the fitness wagon, forgive yourself. Pick yourself up, dust off, and keep moving forward.

NUTRITION

It is impossible to discuss strength training without addressing nutrition. A common saying that you will hear in the gym is "You can't out-train a bad diet." If we continue to consume too many nutrient-empty calories in the form of processed, sugary "foods" without the right balance of macronutrients, our efforts with strength training will end in frustration. For example, a 150-pound person would need to run for about 45 minutes or vigorously lift weights for about 50 minutes to burn 500 calories. It would be infinitely easier to substitute that 500-calorie muffin with an apple, but it's not only about restricting calories for fat loss. Proper nutrition is also about creating the necessary environment to build and strengthen our muscles, which in turn helps increase our metabolic rate.

Micro- and Macronutrients

Micronutrients are vitamins and minerals that our bodies require to remain in good health. They play an important role in human development and wellness, including the regulation of metabolism, heartbeat, and bone density. They can be found in fruits, vegetables, nuts, dairy, and organ meats, among other sources.

Macronutrients are protein, carbohydrates, and fat. A good ratio for building muscle is 25 percent protein, 55 percent carbs, and 20 percent fat, for both men and women. Some nutritionists recommend a ratio of 40 percent carbohydrates, 30 percent protein, and 30 percent fat as a good target for healthy weight loss. To function optimally, our bodies need a good balance of micro- and macronutrients.

Protein

Protein (1 gram = 4 calories) is a key nutrient for gaining strength and size, losing fat, and controlling hunger.

In order to increase muscle mass, the recommendation for active adults is to consume between 1.2 and 1.7 grams of protein per kilogram of your *goal* body weight per day, or 0.5 to 0.8 grams per pound of your goal body weight.

Based on a daily (low) caloric intake of 1500 calories, protein intake should run between 375 and 450 calories, with the higher amount recommended for weight loss. For reference, one chicken thigh contains 13.5 grams of protein and about 110 calories.

Carbohydrates

Carbohydrates (1 gram = 4 calories) often get a bad rap, especially when it comes to weight gain. But carbohydrates aren't all bad. They provide fuel for the brain and energy for our muscles. In general, carbohydrates should make up approximately 40 to 45 percent of your daily caloric intake for weight loss and 55 to 60 percent for maintenance.

It's important to stick with the complex carbohydrates rather than simple carbohydrates. Simple carbohydrates are "foods" with added sugars and refined grains, such as sugary drinks, desserts, and candy, which are packed with useless calories.

Examples of complex carbs are:

» Fiber-rich fruits (raspberries, apples, avocado)
» Vegetables (broccoli, acorn squash, peas, Brussels sprouts)
» Nuts (almonds, pine nuts, pistachios)
» Whole grains (bulgur, barley, amaranth, rye)
» Seeds (chia, flax, sesame)
» Legumes (lima beans, lentils, kidney beans)

Fat

Dietary fat (1 gram = 9 calories) provides energy and helps with nutrient absorption, as well as brain and nerve function. Some unsaturated fatty acids are essential nutrients, meaning that we need to get these fats from food because our bodies can't make them. Fats and oils also add flavor and make you feel full longer and should make up about 20 percent of your daily caloric intake.

The two types of fats are saturated and unsaturated. Saturated fats are solid at room temperature while unsaturated fats are liquid. Unsaturated fats are considered the healthiest type of dietary fat. Choosing unsaturated instead of saturated fats may help reduce your risk of heart disease and stroke.

Pre-Workout Nutrition Ideas

LIGHT MEALS

Depending on the timing of your workout, eating a small meal an hour before your workout may be in order, rather than just an energy snack. Your small meal should be made up of equal parts lean protein and carbs.
   Examples include:

» Two boiled eggs with whole-grain toast and sliced tomatoes
» Whey protein isolate smoothie with fruit, including ½ banana, berries, or apples
» Brown rice or long-grain white rice with half of a chicken breast, or salmon and steamed broccoli
» Small bowl of wheat pasta with tomato and ⅓ cup of meat sauce
» Salad greens, cucumber, tomatoes, bell pepper, dried cranberries with ½ cup of diced chicken
» Whole-grain bagel with smoked salmon, thinly sliced onion, and a thin layer of cream cheese
» Vegan kale Caesar salad with tempeh bacon
» Chicken breast and a stuffed baked potato with asparagus
» Greek salad with half of a grilled chicken breast
» Mediterranean couscous salad with a fresh lemon herb dressing, feta cheese, olives, and chickpeas

SNACKS

Eating lightly around half an hour before your workout will allow you to head in with maximum energy. Combining a complex carbohydrate with a lean protein is the best way to fuel your body.
   Examples include:

» A banana with almond butter
» Multigrain crackers with hummus
» Whole-grain bread with unsweetened peanut butter
» ½ cup of oatmeal with raisins or berries
» Rice cake with peanut butter and sliced apple
» Bowl of plain Greek yogurt with blueberries and granola

Post-Workout Nutrition Ideas

LIGHT MEALS

In general, we want to eat a combination of protein, fats, and carbohydrates before and after our workouts, but our pre-workout should be more carb-dense, and our post-workout nutrition should be more protein-dense.

Examples include:

» Grilled chicken with roasted vegetables
» Two-egg omelet with roasted veggies and whole-grain toast
» 6 ounces of tenderloin steak with brown rice and broccoli
» Salmon with quinoa and green beans
» Prawns, egg pasta noodles, and green salad with oil and vinegar dressing
» Pork tenderloin with roasted veggies and sweet potato
» Avocado and tomato on whole-grain or sourdough toast with Havarti cheese
» Burrito with beans, brown rice, guacamole, and salsa
» Tofu with mushrooms and broccoli
» Chicken salad with mixed greens, tomatoes, bell peppers, onions, and spinach with lemon and olive oil dressing

SNACKS

For those times when you just need to replenish yourself after a workout but aren't ready for a full meal:

» Goat cheese, rice crackers, and olives
» Cottage cheese and fruits
» Pita and hummus
» Protein shake with Greek yogurt and berries
» Handful of almonds or walnuts with goji berries

Hydration

Drinking fluids is crucial to staying healthy for every system in your body. Fluids carry nutrients to your cells, flush bacteria from your bladder, and prevent constipation.

In general, you should drink 16 to 32 ounces of fluid every 60 minutes while exercising. For exercise lasting less than one hour, drink only water. However, if it's excessively hot or humid, a sports drink can be a healthy option. For exercise lasting longer than one hour, drink water, a high-quality sports drink, or both for optimal hydration.

Supplements

First and foremost, do your best to derive nutrients from your foods. However, you may wish to supplement your diet if you suspect you're not getting enough in the food you eat.

B12
Your body uses B12 to fight germs and to make energy. You need more B12 as you get older. It helps your body produce red blood cells, which are responsible for delivering oxygen to the muscles.

Calcium and Magnesium
Together, magnesium and calcium are crucial to bone health. Without magnesium, calcium can become toxic to the kidneys, arteries, and **cartilage**, rather than being deposited in the bones where it's most needed.

Vitamin D
This vitamin helps you absorb calcium, and it can help prevent osteoporosis. It also helps the function of your muscles, nerves, and immune system. Most people get some vitamin D from sunlight, but our body is less able to convert the sun's rays to vitamin D as you age.

Fish Oil
The fatty acids contained in fish oil have several benefits for muscle building, such as reduced muscle soreness. The American Heart Association recommends that people with coronary heart disease take omega-3 fatty acids (the kind found in fish) to prevent heart attacks.

Protein Powder
If you feel that you are having a tough time eating enough protein, you may want to invest in a good protein powder. The various protein powders on the market are a way to ensure that you're getting enough protein to effectively build muscle. There are even some vegan-friendly options on the market. Add a scoop to a smoothie and you'll be good to go!

YOUR GEAR AND YOUR GYM

This book will give you both home workouts that you can do with a few pieces of equipment and workouts that you can do in the gym, if that's your preference. If there are days that you just can't get to the gym or you prefer to exercise at home, it's handy to have two or three varieties of weights and strengths of dumbbells and/or resistance bands.

Some people begin strength training by doing bodyweight exercises at home, and then progressing over time to the use of weights and/or resistance bands. Bodyweight exercises are a great place to start, but remember that your body will not get stronger if you don't progressively add resistance.

Resistance bands

These exercise bands are useful tools for taking your workout with you while traveling. My clients travel a lot and they love taking their bands with them on their adventures in order to keep their strength up while away. Band exercises are surprisingly effective and inexpensive. Anything you can do with dumbbells, you can do with these bands.

Dumbbells

If working out at home, please refer to chapter 5 for weight suggestions. You may soon find that you are back at the sporting goods store looking for heavier dumbbells as your body gets stronger. Basically, you will use the lighter weights for your smaller muscles (like arms and shoulders) and the heavier weights for your larger muscles (like your chest, back, and legs).

Shoes

For both home and gym, be sure you have a pair of good athletic shoes. I am a fan of the lighter sports shoes rather than the very thick-soled, heavy athletic shoes that you can find on the market. However, if you have foot issues and have been specifically advised by your doctor, be sure to follow their advice regarding footwear. If you are a runner and own specific running shoes, feel free to wear those while you lift weights.

Water bottle

I suggest you keep a refillable water bottle with you while you're exercising and throughout the day. That way you can keep track of your hydration and avoid potential dehydration or even heat exhaustion.

Gloves

You also may want to invest in a pair of durable weightlifting gloves to keep your palms callous-free.

REST AND RECOVERY

You may hear about the importance of exercise and the negative effects of inactivity, but it's not as common to hear about why you also need to allow your body time to rest. Resting is equally as important as working out for building muscle.

Rest

Getting enough rest between workouts allows your muscles the opportunity to rebuild and regenerate before your next session. The recommended amount of rest time between strength sessions targeting the same muscle groups is 48 hours. But "rest" doesn't mean that we don't move at all. On your days off, go for a nice long walk, attend a Zumba class, or do some restorative yoga.

Sleep

Rapid eye movement (REM) sleep is crucial for strength training recovery, since it is during this time that protein synthesis and human growth hormones are released, allowing for muscle repair and recovery.

With too little sleep, the body is more likely to produce the stress hormone cortisol. I won't get into the science of it all, but *know* that studies have shown that there is a definite connection between lack of sleep and the elevation of cortisol levels, which can contribute to atrophy in both muscle and bone, as well as weight gain.

How to Evaluate Need for Recovery

After a good strength training workout, expect to feel some muscle soreness the next day or even two days later. This is called delayed onset muscle soreness (DOMS). Rest assured you won't always be feeling muscle soreness; but in the beginning, when you push harder, or when you change up your program, you will probably feel some muscle soreness. This is all normal and perfectly safe.

However, if you're feeling *excessive* fatigue after a workout, you may have pushed too hard. If that happens, simply go a little easier next time. Get your rest, proper nutrition, adequate sleep, and keep going.

GET PUMPED: GOAL WORKSHEET

I often tell my clients that if they are to be successful with maintaining their strength training motivation, it is imperative to find their "*Why.*" I explain the difference between inspiration and motivation by saying that inspiration comes from outside of oneself, while motivation comes from within.

Consider asking yourself any of the following, if you are in search of your motivation:

» How do I want to interact with my children/grandchildren? Do I want to be enjoying the ski slopes or the ocean with them rather than always sitting on the sidelines as a spectator?

» How do I see my future travels? Am I willing to settle for not being able to climb the hill to see the view, scramble around the ruins, or keep up with the tour?

» Am I willing to allow weakened joints to sideline me from my favorite hikes and sports?

» I've heard that strength training will help me with my depression/anxiety/mood. Am I willing to try everything I can to elevate my mood naturally?

» I've heard that strength training helps with cognitive health. Am I willing to do whatever I can to maintain a healthy brain?

» I want to maintain an active and fun sex life, but am I willing to risk losing that by not maintaining my strength and my vital energy?

MASTER THE MOVES

In this chapter you will find tutorials on how to do the exercises (with variations) within the workouts in chapters 4 through 9. You may want to look them over and give them a trial run prior to week 1. Please refer to these pages until you have mastered each exercise.

DYNAMIC STRETCHES (WARM-UP)

Dynamic stretches are active movements where joints and muscles go through a full range of motion. They are best used to prepare your body for exercise. Some examples of dynamic warm-up movements include:

» Leg swings (side to side and front to back)
» Arm rotations
» Marching in place while pumping arms
» Jumping jacks
» Hip circles
» Mountain climbers

Dynamic stretches are activities which involve movement, whereas static stretches (described in the next section) are positions where muscles are extended and held for 15 to 30 seconds. Static stretches should never be used as a warm-up to exercise.

If you have access to cardio equipment, feel free to use it for warming up instead of the dynamic movements. If the cardio equipment you choose does not involve your upper body, be sure to add movements such as arm and shoulder rotations.

STATIC STRETCHES (COOLDOWN)

Our muscles are not in charge of our range of motion. They facilitate bone and joint actions, which determine range of motion. Studies have shown that by continuously performing intense stretches and pushing beyond our natural range of motion, we may be creating uneven wear and tear on the joints and ligaments, which can lead to osteoarthritis.

While we don't want to stretch beyond what is natural for us, most people don't hold stretches for long enough. As I previously mentioned, we want to hold static stretches for 15 to 30 seconds, but remember it isn't supposed to hurt. Concentrating on steady breathing will help deliver more oxygen to and remove more waste products from the muscle fibers.

The following stretches are a great way to cool down *after* your workout and can be performed on your "off" days as well, to help maintain the range of motion that is optimal for *your* body.

THE EXERCISES

The home workouts include bodyweight exercises, dumbbell exercises, and resistance band variations. You should have two bands of different strengths on hand prior to week 2 for the home workouts. If you would like to add more options to your workout, you will find a variety of dumbbells at most sporting goods stores. You may want to consider purchasing dumbbells in two different weights (see page 157 for dumbbell weight guidelines). In general, you will use the lighter bands and weights for the smaller muscle groups, and you will use the heavier bands and weights for the larger muscles, such as those in your legs.

Gym workouts include dumbbells, bodyweight, gym machines, and a stability ball. Most gyms will have this equipment available for you.

Regardless of the equipment you use, proper form is imperative, so that you target the correct muscles and remain injury-free. For every exercise, use controlled motions in both phases: the lifting and lowering back down. Quick, jerky motions can lead to injury. Slow down and concentrate on what you're doing, and on the muscles you're targeting. Remember, it's not supposed to be easy, but that doesn't mean it can't be fun!

muscle groups

Quadriceps

QUADRICEPS STRETCH

To properly stretch all your quad muscles, you'll have to not only bend your knee but stand up straight enough to feel the stretch in the front of the hip of the standing leg.

INSTRUCTIONS

1. While standing on a straight leg, hold on to a countertop or chair back to assist in balance.

2. Bend your other knee back by grasping your ankle with one hand.

3. Assist in bending your knee back as far as possible, gently pressing your foot toward your glutes. If this causes stress on your knees, be very gentle.

4. Push the hips forward to engage slightly so that you engage the hip flexors (the front of your hips, where your legs meet your torso). Hold for 15 to 30 seconds (don't forget to breathe).

5. Return to a standing position. Repeat with the opposite leg.

6. Repeat two to three times on both sides.

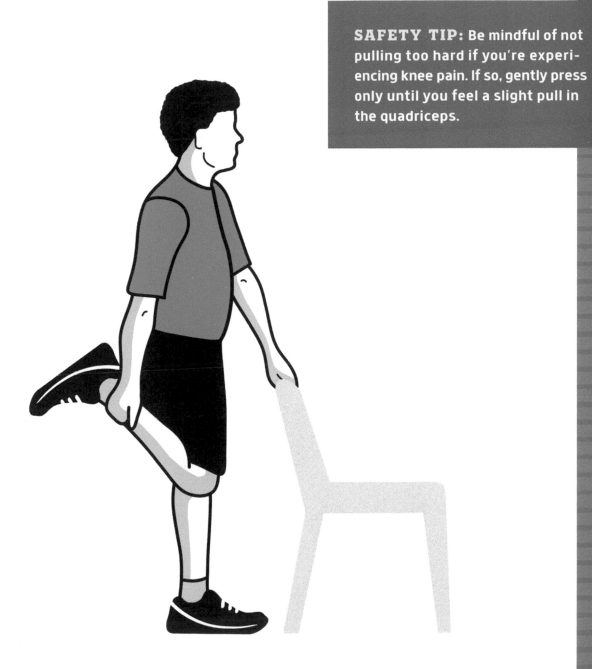

muscle groups

Hamstrings

HAMSTRING STRETCH

It is especially important to give the hamstrings a good stretch prior to exercise. Tight hamstrings may be more prone to strain or tearing.

INSTRUCTIONS

1. Avoid throwing the leg up onto a high elevation.

2. Gently place your heel onto a chair-height surface, keeping both legs straight.

3. Your spine should be kept as straight as possible while bending forward at the hips.

4. Bring the torso toward your leg, without curving your spine. Hold for 15 to 30 seconds. (Don't forget to breathe.)

5. Repeat with the opposite leg.

6. Feel free to repeat two to three times.

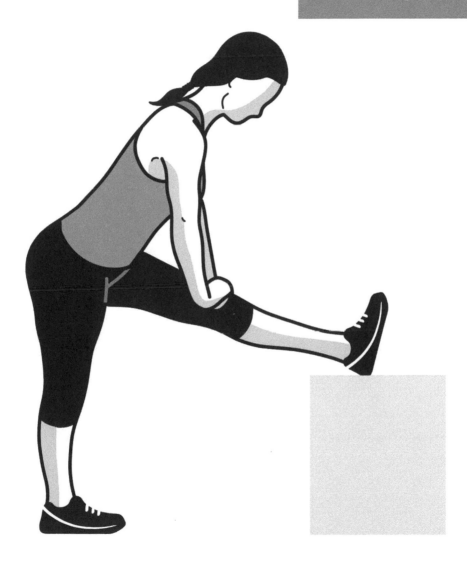

STATIC STRETCHES

muscle groups

Adductors

Groin

INNER THIGH STRETCH

This stretch protects the hips by helping maintain and improve outward rotation in the hips.

INSTRUCTIONS

1. Sit with your feet together, hips turned out, knees bent, back straight, chin level.

2. Bring your feet in as close to your body as you can while allowing the knees to splay out comfortably.

3. Keeping your back straight, gently lean forward from the hips until you feel a slight stretching sensation along the inner thighs.

4. Rest your elbows on your knees to hold the position for 15 to 30 seconds. Breathe.

5. Relax completely before repeating the steps two to three times.

SAFETY TIP: Do not bounce your legs. Simply press gently and hold.

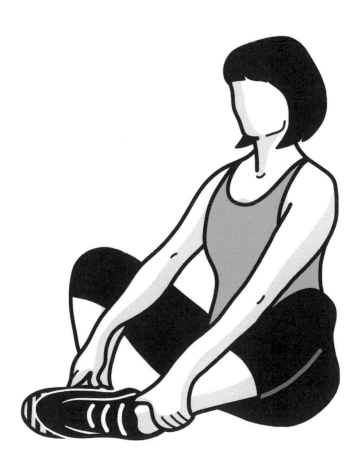

muscle groups

Gastrocnemius

Soleus

CALF STRETCH

These muscles play a major role in walking and running, and any level of tightness can lead to pain and imbalance in other areas of your body. It's particularly important to stretch your calf muscles if you wear high heels often or if you sit at a desk for long periods of time.

INSTRUCTIONS

1. Begin by standing two to three feet away from a wall, depending on your height.

2. Place one foot in front of your body as you lean toward the wall.

3. Rest your hands up against the wall at about chest height. Keep your heels, hips, and head in a straight line and your feet flat on the floor.

4. Lean forward while pressing your rear heel into the floor, until you feel a stretch in your calves. Hold for 15 to 30 seconds. (Don't forget to breathe.)

5. To stretch the soleus, come away from the wall, standing more upright.

6. Gently bend the back leg until you feel the stretch lower down toward your heel. Hold for 15 to 30 seconds.

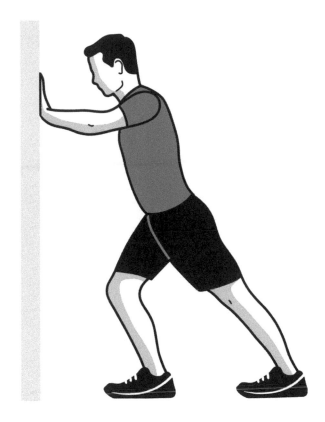

SAFETY TIP: Avoid this stretch if you are experiencing Achilles tendon issues.

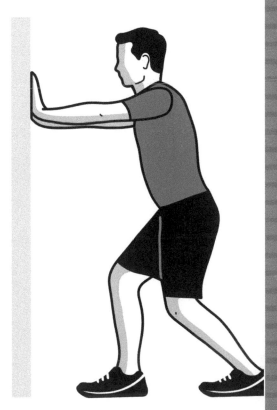

muscle groups

Latissimus Dorsi

BACK STRETCH

The latissimus dorsi are the large, broad muscles located on each side of your upper and mid back.

INSTRUCTIONS

1. Find a ledge that is approximately chest height, such as a fireplace mantle, or simply place your hands on a wall at the same height.

2. Place your hands shoulder-width apart. Without moving your arms, slowly bend forward at your hips. Allow your head to drop toward your chest.

3. Stop when you feel a stretch along the sides of your upper and mid back. (Don't forget to breathe.) Hold for 15 to 30 seconds, and then relax.

4. Repeat two to three times.

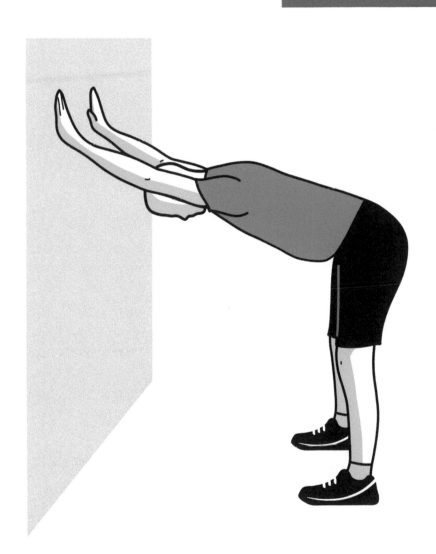

muscle groups

Pectoralis Major

Pectoralis Minor

Anterior Deltoid

CHEST STRETCH

One of the most important muscle groups to stretch is the pectoralis muscles, more commonly known as the chest muscles.

INSTRUCTIONS

1. Stand at the right angle of two walls or in a doorway.

2. Place your left arm at 90 degrees onto the doorjamb or edge of the wall. Gently rotate your body away from that arm, away from the working side.

3. You may have to shift your feet slightly, to point away from working side. Also, you may need to rotate the non-working shoulder back a little in order to feel the stretch. (You should feel the stretch in the front of the working-side armpit.)

4. Hold for 15 to 30 seconds on each side. (Don't forget to breathe.)

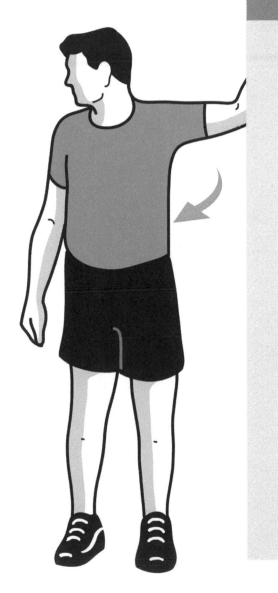

SAFETY TIP: Use caution as you rotate your torso away from the contact point.

STATIC STRETCHES

muscle groups

Quadratus Lumborum ▶

LOWER BACK STRETCH

The quadratus lumborum is the deepest abdominal muscle and is located in your lower back, on either side of the lumbar spine.

INSTRUCTIONS

1. From a standing position, place one hand on your hip and raise the other arm over your head.

2. Bend to the side, extending your raised arm and reaching over toward the opposite side. (You can adjust where the stretch hits by reaching slightly in front of your body.)

3. Tuck in your chin and gaze down toward the floor. Hold this position for 15 to 30 seconds. (Don't forget to breathe.)

4. Repeat on the other side.

5. To deepen the stretch, hold one wrist with your opposite hand as you stretch, or cross one leg in front of the other.

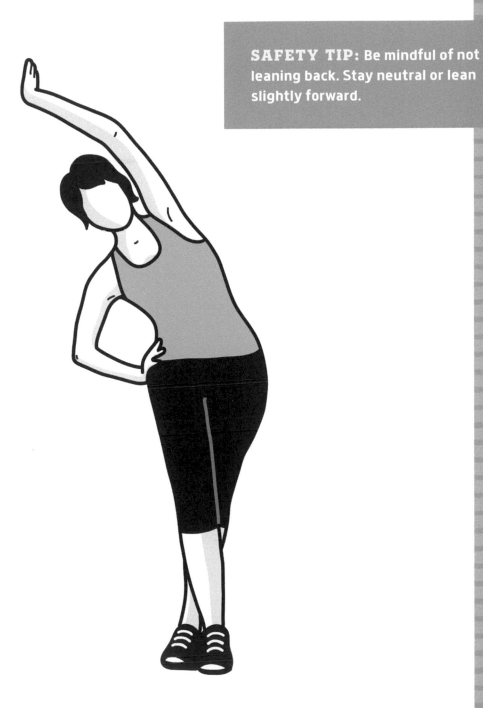

SAFETY TIP: Be mindful of not leaning back. Stay neutral or lean slightly forward.

muscle groups

Piriformis

DEEP HIP STRETCH

If the piriformis pushes against the sciatic nerve (often caused by too much sitting), it can cause excruciating pain.

INSTRUCTIONS

1. Lie on your back, bend both knees, and bring your left ankle over your right thigh.

2. Lift your right foot off the ground, bringing your leg up to a 90-degree angle.

3. Loop your hands in between your legs and slowly draw your right knee in toward your chest.

4. Keep your head and neck relaxed on the ground, holding for 15 to 30 seconds. (Don't forget to breathe.)

5. Repeat on the other side.

6. You can also do this stretch in a seated position by placing your ankle on the opposite knee and leaning forward until you feel that stretch deep in the back of your hip.

SAFETY TIP: If you're doing the seated version, be careful not to curve your spine forward. Keep your back flat as you lean forward.

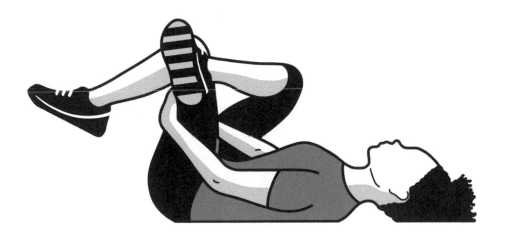

Static Stretch Program (Cooldown)

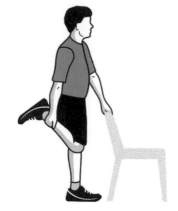

QUADRICEPS STRETCH
PAGE 24

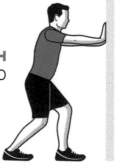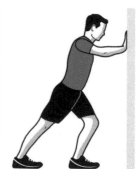

CALF STRETCH
PAGE 30

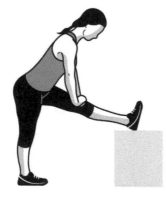

HAMSTRING STRETCH
PAGE 26

INNER THIGH STRETCH
PAGE 28

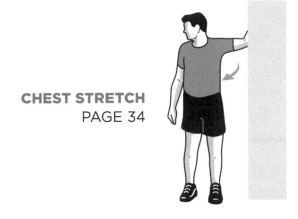

CHEST STRETCH
PAGE 34

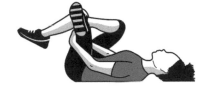

DEEP HIP STRETCH
PAGE 38

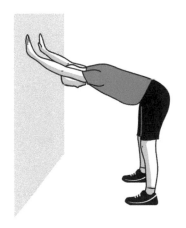

BACK STRETCH
PAGE 32

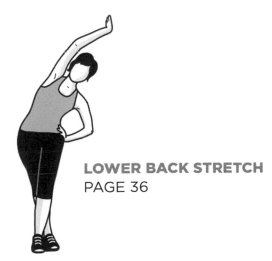

LOWER BACK STRETCH
PAGE 36

BODYWEIGHT EXERCISES

Bodyweight exercises are a great way to start with strength training, though they have limitations due to the challenges of adding resistance. There are ways, however, of modifying bodyweight exercises over time to make them more difficult. For example, you can add time to the plank, add repetitions to all exercises, and slow the movements down.

muscle groups

Rectus Abdominis

Spinal Erectors

Transverse Abdominis

FOREARM PLANK

The plank is an essential core strength building exercise for any level. The goal is to hold the position for a set length of time, or for as long as possible without dropping or lifting the hips.

INSTRUCTIONS

1. Make a straight line from your shoulders to your heels, keeping your neck neutral by looking down.

2. Keep your elbows beneath your shoulders. Stay relaxed and breathe.

3. Hold for as long as you can (up to 60 seconds).

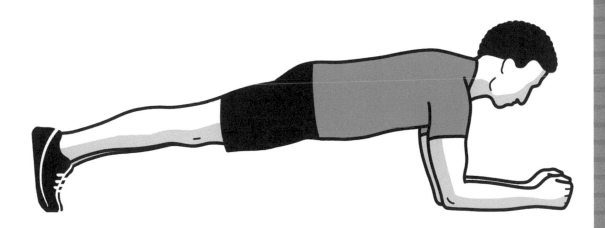

muscle groups

Rectus Abdominis
(with focus on the lower portion)

PARTIAL CRUNCH

Partial crunches are superior to the sit-up because they utilize the portion of a sit-up where the muscles are fully engaged.

INSTRUCTIONS

1. Lie on your back with your knees bent and feet flat on the floor.

2. Place your hands behind your head. It's best not to lace your fingers together. You may also cross your arms at your chest if that's more comfortable.

3. Gently pull your abdominals inward.

4. Curl up and forward so that your head, neck, and shoulders lift off the floor.

5. Aim for two sets of 10 to 15 repetitions.

6. For more of a challenge, hold the legs up at 90 degrees while you perform the exercise.

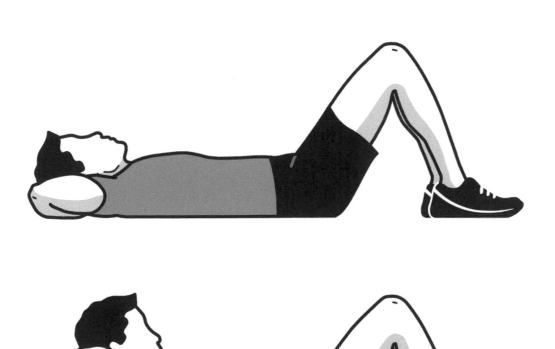

muscle groups

Rectus Abdominis
(with focus on the lower portion)

REVERSE CRUNCH

The reverse crunch is a popular exercise which targets the abdominals, particularly the lower portion.

INSTRUCTIONS

1. Lie flat on your back with your hands beneath your hips.

2. Bend your knees and lift them toward your head, keeping the knees bent at 90 degrees.

3. Draw them upward slightly at the end of the movement. Be careful to not use momentum to swing your legs overhead. Concentrate on your abdominal muscles acting like an accordion to "fold" your bent legs up over your torso.

4. For a more advanced version, try to lift your hips off the floor as your legs are at the top of the movement. If you cannot do this, with constant effort, as your core gets stronger, you may find that you can lift your hips off the floor.

5. Lower your feet back down just above the floor, without fully extending your legs, to complete one repetition. Repeat to the desired number of reps.

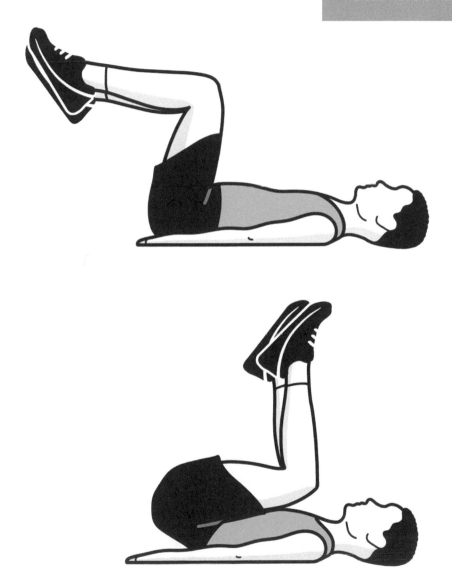

muscle groups

Spinal Erectors

Transverse Abdominis

DEAD BUG

The dead bug might seem quite easy for the first couple of repetitions, but if you keep your core engaged, by pressing the lower back into the floor you will feel the fatigue soon enough.

INSTRUCTIONS

1. Lie flat on your back with your arms extended toward the ceiling.

2. Bring your legs up so your knees are bent at 90-degree angles. This is your starting position.

3. Slowly lower your right arm and left leg at the same time, until your arm and leg are just above the floor. The arm and leg should be straight and fully extended.

4. Then slowly return to the starting position, keeping the arm extended and bending the leg back to 90 degrees. Repeat with the opposite limbs.

5. Use slow controlled motions when lowering and returning to the starting position. Be sure your back is flat against the floor throughout the movement.

6. Aim for 10 repetitions on each side. Work up to two rounds of this exercise.

7. For a more advanced version of the dead bug, keep your shoulders off the floor throughout the movement and be mindful of keeping the bent knee at 90 degrees (the thigh of the non-extended leg should be perpendicular to the floor).

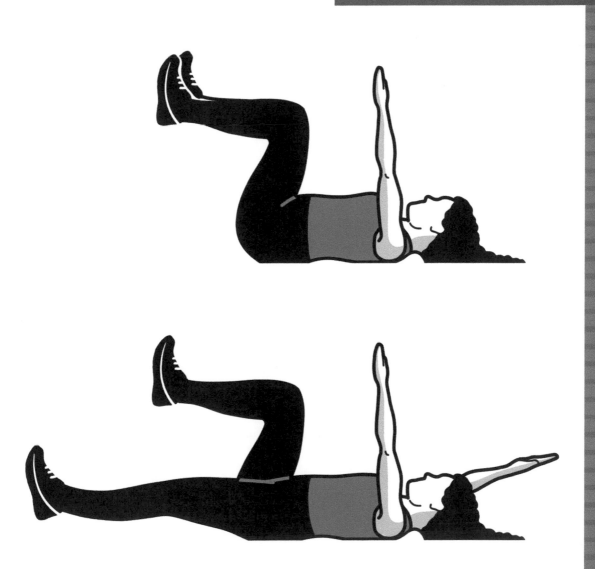

muscle groups

External Obliques

Internal Obliques

Transverse Abdominis

Quadratus Lumborum

SIDE PLANK

This exercise targets a host of muscles which act as stabilizers.

INSTRUCTIONS

1. Lie on your side with your forearm flat on the floor, bottom elbow lined up directly under your shoulder, and both legs either extended out in a long line or bent at 90 degrees for an easier modification. Your top hand can be on the side of your hip (easier) or reaching up to the ceiling (more challenging).

2. If legs are extended, feet can either be staggered for more stability or stacked for more of a challenge.

3. For an intermediate version, keep your bottom leg bent but extend your top leg out, actively engaging your inner thigh as you push your top leg into the floor.

4. Engage your core and lift your hips off the floor, forming a straight line from your head to your feet, or from head to knees for the modification. Keep hips pressed upward. You should feel this mostly on the side closest to the floor.

5. Hold for 15 to 30 seconds and build up to 60 seconds over time.

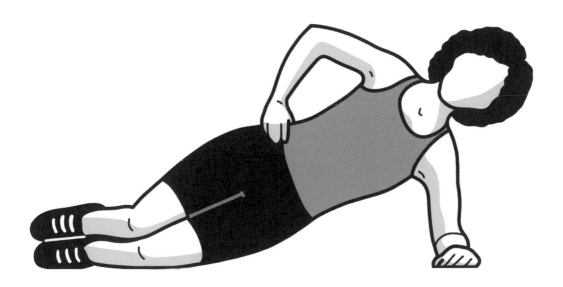

muscle groups

Pectoralis Major

Pectoralis Minor

Anterior Deltoid

PUSH-UP (WITH VARIATIONS)

Push-Ups from Knees (Easier)

The more parallel to the floor our body is, the more challenging the move. Therefore, a chair push-up is more challenging than a table-height push-up. A push-up from your knees is easier than one from the toes.

INSTRUCTIONS

1. Start in high plank with your shoulders, elbows, and wrists stacked and your spine long.

2. Come down onto your knees. Your body should be in a straight line from knees to head.

3. Bend your elbows and lower your chest to the ground.

4. Push through the palms of your hands to straighten your arms.

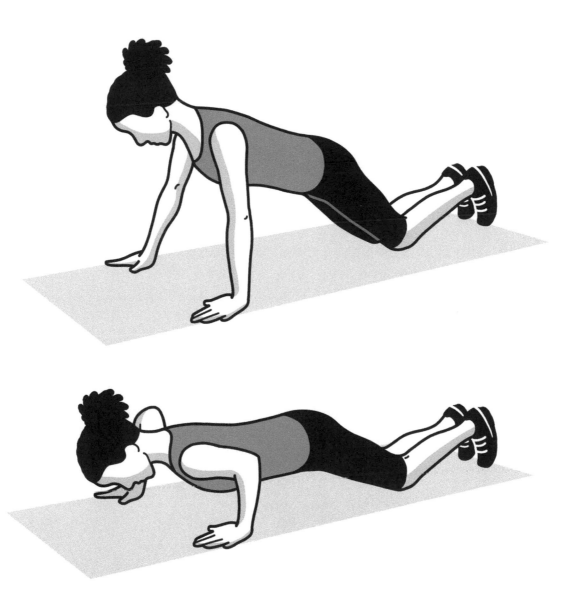

BODYWEIGHT EXERCISES

Push-Ups from Table/Chair (Medium Challenge)

You can adjust the degree of challenge by varying the degree of your body. At home, some handy objects to use are a table or chair. Be sure the objects you're using are stable. You don't want them to move out from under you. Keep your body in a straight line as you lower and push back up.

INSTRUCTIONS

1. Position an object, such as a chair, with its back against a wall.

2. Grasp both sides of the chair seat and move your feet back until you are aligned from the tip of your head to your feet.

3. Engage your core by pulling your belly button inward.

4. Lower your chest toward the chair as far as you comfortably can, while still maintaining your form. Avoid letting your elbow curve outward.

5. Push back up while maintaining your body alignment. Return to the starting position and repeat to the desired reps.

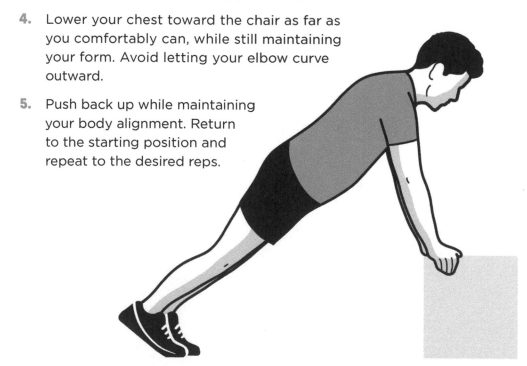

Push-Ups from Toes with Brief Rest Stop (More Challenging)

Fully extending your legs increases the difficulty of this move by adding more body weight.

INSTRUCTIONS

1. Begin with your chest and stomach flat on the floor. Your legs should be straight out behind you with toes tucked. Your palms should be at chest level with the arms bent out at a 45-degree angle.

2. Exhale as you push from your hands and heels, bringing your entire body off the floor.

3. Pause for a second in the straight-arm plank position, keeping your core engaged.

4. Inhale as you slowly lower back to your starting position.

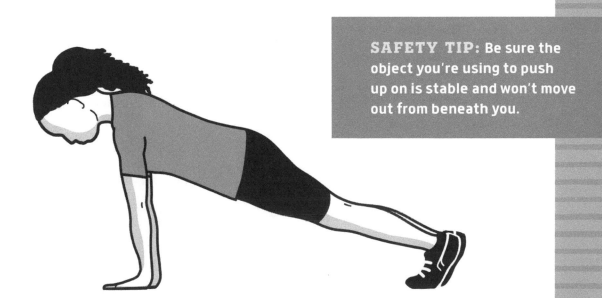

SAFETY TIP: Be sure the object you're using to push up on is stable and won't move out from beneath you.

muscle groups

Anterior Deltoid

Pectoralis Major

Pectoralis Minor

Triceps

TRICEPS DIP (WITH VARIATIONS)

The triceps dip is an amazing exercise for anyone looking to strengthen the back of their upper arms, not only for aesthetic reasons but for added strength for any kind of pushing motion.

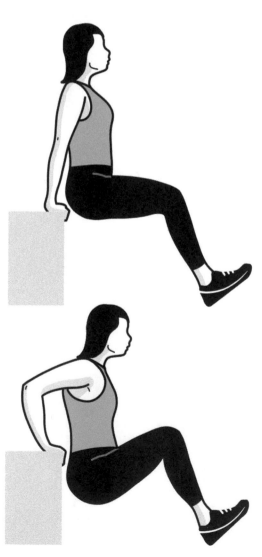

Bent Legs (Easier)

INSTRUCTIONS

1. Sit on the edge of one chair or bench and grip the edge with your hands.

2. Place your heels on the edge of the other chair and hold yourself up using your triceps.

3. Slide forward just far enough that your behind clears the edge of the chair, then lower yourself until your elbows are bent as close to 90 degrees as possible.

4. Push back up until your arms are straight, without using your legs to assist in pushing.

Straight Leg (More Challenging)

INSTRUCTIONS

1. Grasp the front edge of a chair-height object near your thighs.

2. Walk your feet forward until the hips are slightly bent, with your legs straight arms extended.

3. Bend the elbows to about 90 degrees and lower your hips toward the floor.

4. Push back up to starting position. Be careful not to lock out the elbows for too long, as this serves as a rest.

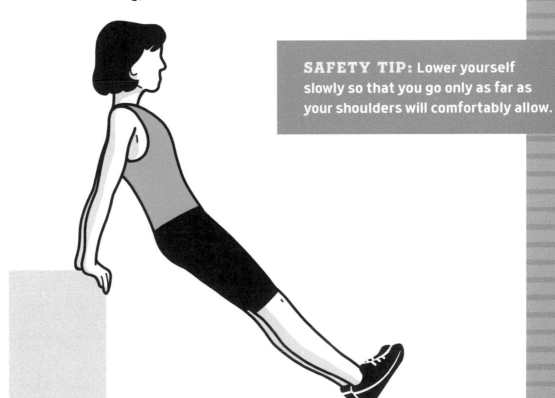

SAFETY TIP: Lower yourself slowly so that you go only as far as your shoulders will comfortably allow.

muscle groups

Spinal Erectors

Abdominals
(to a lesser degree)

Glutes
(to a lesser degree)

Hamstrings
(to a lesser degree)

BIRD DOG

The bird dog engages both the core and back muscles at the same time. It is regarded as a safe exercise during recovery from a back injury.

INSTRUCTIONS

1. Begin on all fours with your hands directly under your shoulders and your knees directly under your hips.

2. Pull your abs into your spine. Keeping your back and pelvis still and stable, reach your right arm forward and left leg back. Don't allow the pelvis to rock side to side as you move your leg behind you. Focus on not letting the rib cage sag toward the floor. Reach through your left heel to engage the muscles in the back of the leg and your glutes.

3. Return to the starting position, placing your hand and knee on the floor. Repeat on the other side to complete one rep.

4. Work up to 10 to 12 reps on each side.

TIP: Try to keep your hips square to the floor as you alternate limb extensions.

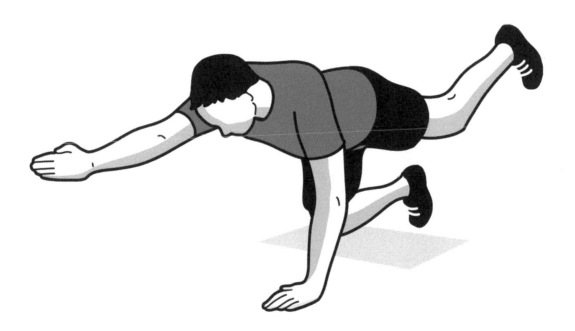

muscle groups

Glutes

Quadriceps

BODYWEIGHT CHAIR SQUATS OR FREESTANDING SQUATS

The squat is a fundamental movement that strengthens the lower body. It's important for beginners to learn proper form before progressing to weighted (dumbbells, barbell) squats.

INSTRUCTIONS

1. Set your feet shoulder-width apart, toes slightly turned out.

2. Initiate the movement by pushing your hips back first. (Like you're shutting the car door with your glutes because your hands are full.)

3. Slowly bend at the knees, continuing to push your hips back until your thighs are as close to parallel to the floor as possible.

4. At the bottom of the movement, pause for a second or two and strongly push back up to the starting position. Keep your chin parallel to the floor and keep your back straight.

5. Repeat to the desired number of reps.

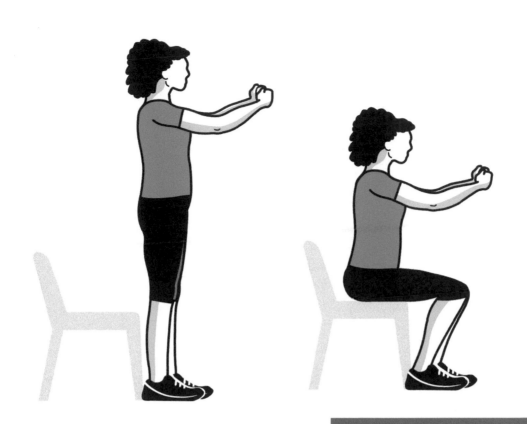

TIP: If you find the freestanding squats too difficult at first, use the chair to rest for a second before pushing back up. Progress to the freestanding version as soon as you comfortably can.

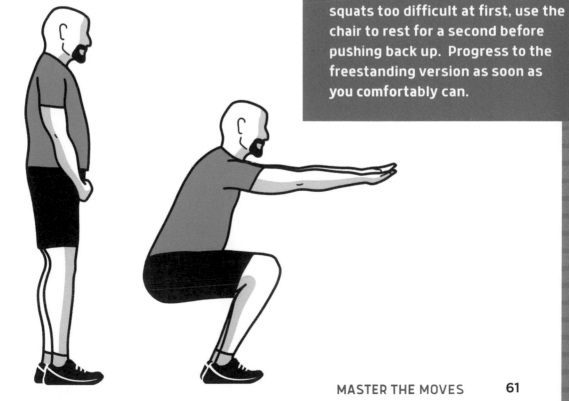

muscle groups

Glutes

Quadriceps

SINGLE-LEG SQUAT TO CHAIR OR BENCH (ADVANCED)

The single-leg squat is an advanced alternative to the basic bodyweight or chair squat, which requires no equipment. The bench or chair will serve as a resting place before pushing back up. But don't sit down for too long.

INSTRUCTIONS

1. Stand in front of a weight bench or chair and lift one leg slightly in front of you. The lower the resting spot is, the harder this will be.

2. Push your hips back and squat down to the bench.

3. Try to barely touch down before rising back up to a standing position. Your free foot will extend more toward the floor as you come up but will naturally come forward as you lower.

4. Push through your heel into the floor as you rise back to a standing position. Avoid swinging your arms to help you get back up.

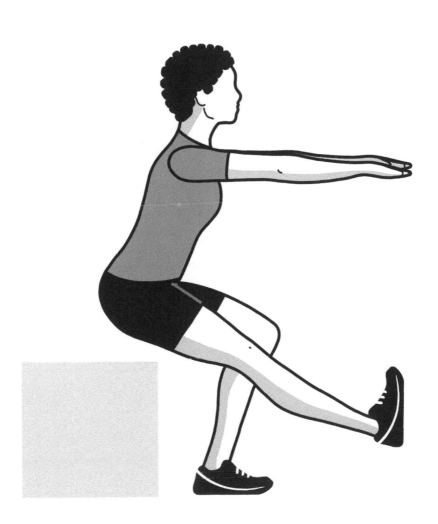

muscle groups

Glutes

Quadriceps

SPLIT SQUATS (WITH BODYWEIGHT OR DUMBBELLS)

The split squat targets the same leg muscles as the squat but places additional tension on the core, knees, and hips, which helps with overall functional strength.

INSTRUCTIONS

1. If you are using dumbbells, be sure to have them in hand, with arms hanging down by your side.

2. From a standing position, take a long step forward as if performing a lunge. The heel of your back foot should be raised.

3. Keeping your torso upright, lower slowly until your back knee almost touches the floor, and the front thigh is as close to parallel as possible.

4. Push back up through the heel of your front foot.

5. Complete all your reps on one leg and then switch to the other.

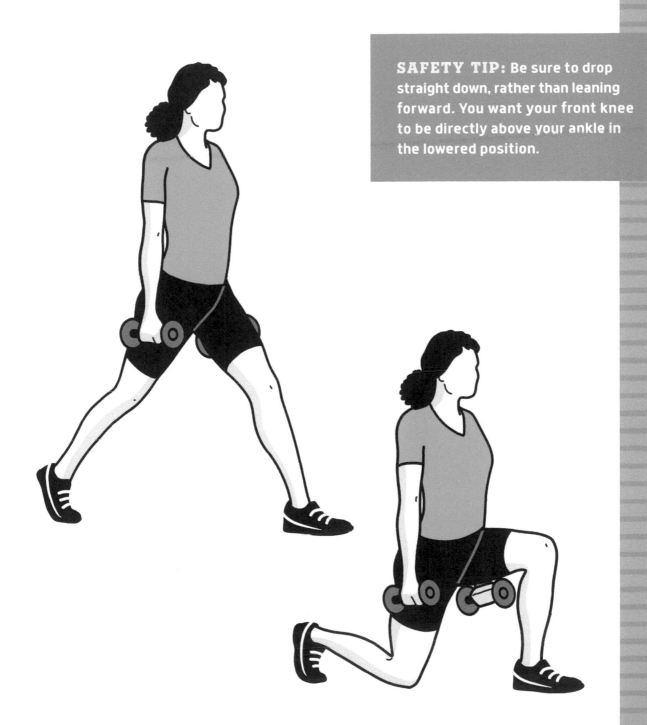

muscle groups

Abdominal

Glutes

Hamstrings

GLUTE BRIDGE

The gluteus maximus (often referred to as the glutes) is the largest of your muscles and helps push you into a standing position and supports your low back.

INSTRUCTIONS

1. Bend your knees and put your feet flat on the ground, just close enough so that you can graze your heels with your fingertips when you stretch your arms down by your side. Your feet should be about hip-width apart.

2. To make the exercise a little more challenging, bend your elbows to 90 degrees so that only your upper arms are on the ground, and forearms are pointing to the ceiling. Otherwise, place arms flat on the floor at about a 45-degree angle from your body.

3. Drive up through your heels and upper back to lift your glutes off the ground. Drive your hips up as high as possible, squeezing the glutes hard. Do not push backward off your heels. Make sure you are driving straight up and that your knees aren't caving in.

4. Squeeze your glutes for a second or two at the top and lower all the way back down to the ground before repeating to the desired number of reps.

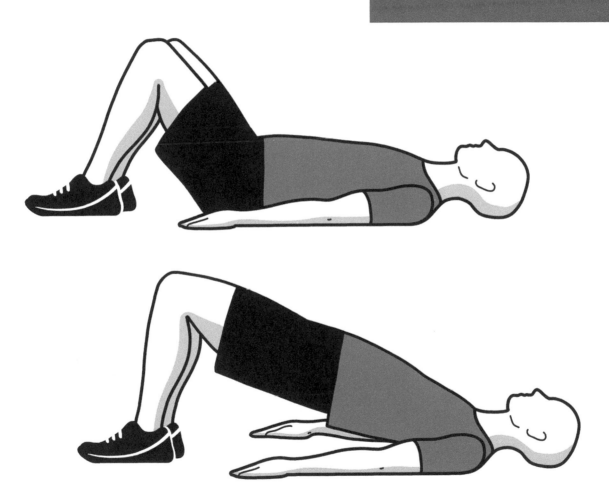

muscle groups

Abdominal

Glutes

Hamstrings

SINGLE-LEG GLUTE BRIDGE (ON FLOOR OR BENCH)

This exercise can be done on the floor or with your upper back on a weight bench at the gym.

INSTRUCTIONS

1. Set up like you would for the glute bridge and then raise one leg up off the ground.

2. You can bend the raised leg to 90 degrees or point the toe up toward the ceiling. Just make sure not to swing the raised leg as you lift.

3. Drive up through your heels and upper back, lifting your hips as high as you can.

4. Hold at the top and then lower back down.

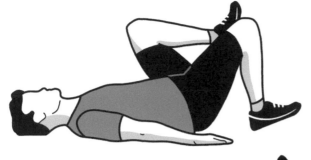

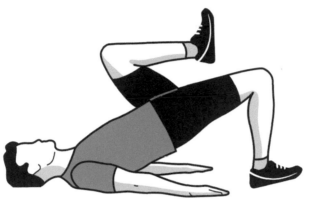

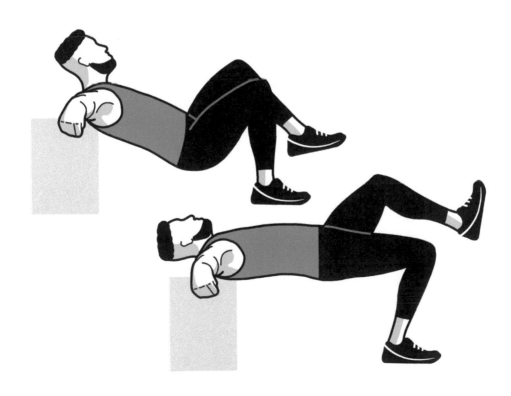

DUMBBELL (FREE WEIGHT) EXERCISES

You will find dumbbells in any gym, but you can also purchase them and use them at home. They are relatively inexpensive and can be easily stored under a sofa or bed. Having as few as two or three sets of dumbbells greatly increases your home strength training options. You can also find adjustable versions, which allow you to quickly change the load, giving a wide range of options.

muscle groups

Biceps

Latissimus Dorsi

Rhomboids

BENT-OVER ROW

A classic among exercises that build back strength, the bent-over row is a must in your workout routine, whether with dumbbells, a barbell, or a resistance band.

INSTRUCTIONS

1. Begin the movement by placing your feet at shoulder width and your toes pointed slightly out.

2. Bend slightly at the knees and forward at the hips. Maintain a braced core and flat back throughout.

3. Leading with your elbows, pull the dumbbells back, bringing your shoulder blades closer together. Hold this contraction and slowly release to the starting position.

4. Slowly lower the dumbbells. Repeat.

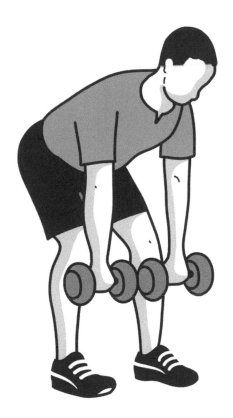

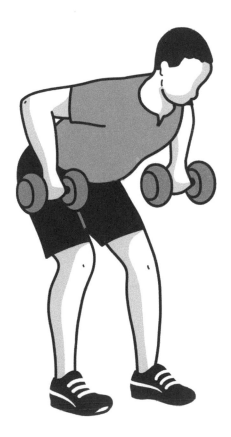

DUMBBELL (FREE WEIGHT) EXERCISES

muscle groups

Pectoralis Major

Pectoralis Minor

Triceps

CHEST PRESS: FLOOR OR COFFEE TABLE (HOME) OR BENCH (GYM)

Use the weight that fatigues your muscles in the 12-repetition range. If you have a piece of furniture that can mimic the weight bench, feel free to use that; otherwise, lie flat on the floor with your legs fully extended or bent with feet on the floor.

INSTRUCTIONS

1. Lie on the floor, bench, or furniture with a dumbbell in each hand.

2. Begin with your arms fully extended.

3. Slowly lower the dumbbells until your arms are at 90 degrees. If you're on the floor, the backs of your upper arms should barely brush the floor (do not rest down).

4. Push the dumbbells back up until the arms are straight.

5. Arch the weights together at the top of the movement. Repeat.

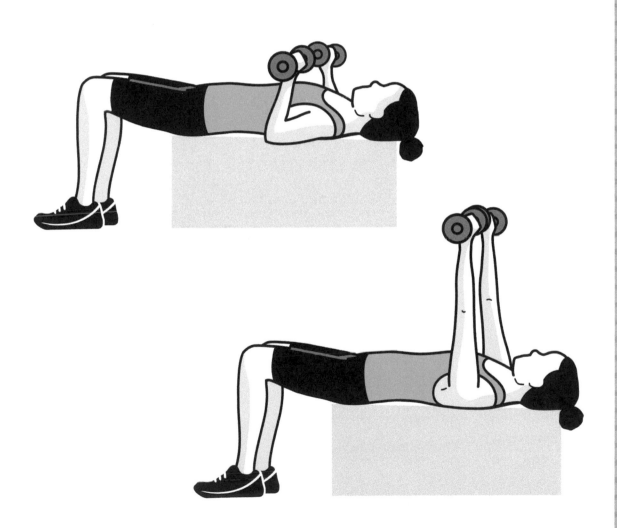

DUMBBELL (FREE WEIGHT) EXERCISES

muscle groups

Anterior Deltoid

Pectoralis Major

Pectoralis Minor

INCLINE CHEST PRESS ON BENCH (GYM)

This exercise targets the upper portion of the chest. The incline press also hits the anterior head of the deltoid muscle of the shoulders, or the front part of your shoulder a little more than the flat-bench version.

INSTRUCTIONS

1. Set the incline of the incline bench at about 30 degrees.

2. Pick up the dumbbells off the floor using a neutral grip, with your palms facing inward. Position the ends of the dumbbells in your hip crease and sit down on the edge of the bench.

3. To get into position, lie back and keep the weights close to your chest. Once you are in position, take a deep breath, and press the dumbbells toward the ceiling until your arms are fully extended.

4. Slowly lower the dumbbells with control as far as comfortably possible (the dumbbells should be about level with your chest).

5. Contract the chest and push the dumbbells back up to the starting position.

6. Repeat to the desired number of reps.

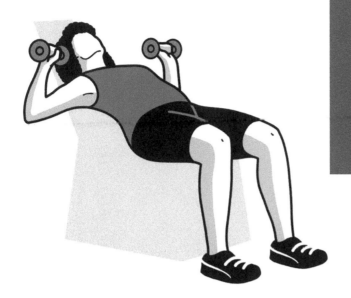

SAFETY TIP: Clutch the dumbbells close to your belly and sit upright in between sets and when you're done. Avoid getting into the habit of dropping them on the floor while lying down, which can be very hard on the shoulder joints.

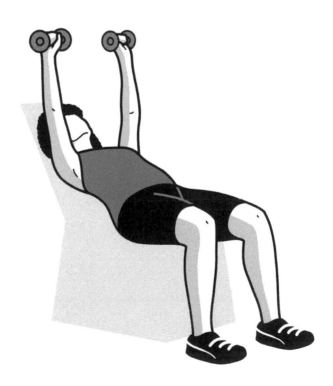

DUMBBELL (FREE WEIGHT) EXERCISES

muscle groups

Medial Deltoid

LATERAL SHOULDER RAISE

The lateral raise is an upper body isolation exercise for building shoulder strength. This exercise focuses on the medial head of the deltoid and can be done with dumbbells or a resistance band.

INSTRUCTIONS

1. Stand with your feet together or hip-distance apart, with slightly bent knees.

2. Begin with your arms by your sides with your palms facing inward. You may bring your arms in front of you so that the dumbbells are almost touching.

3. Keeping your arms straight, slowly raise your arms to the sides until they're shoulder height and parallel to the floor.

4. Slowly return to the starting position and repeat using slow, controlled motions.

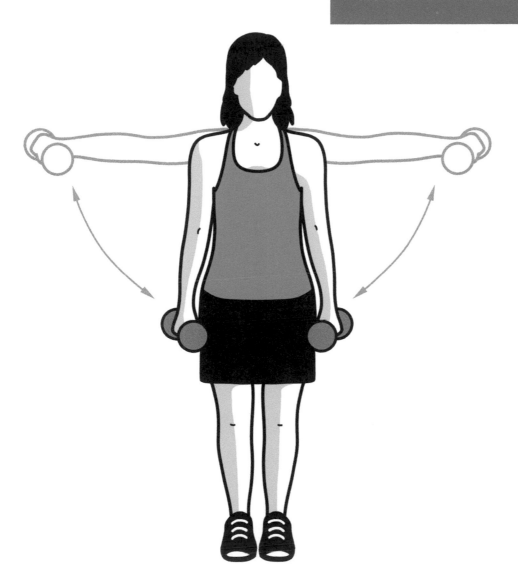

TIP: Keep your elbows slightly bent throughout the motion. The elbow joint does not move whatsoever for the duration of the exercise.

DUMBBELL (FREE WEIGHT) EXERCISES

muscle groups

Deltoids

Pectoralis Major

Pectoralis Minor

Trapezius

Triceps

STANDING OR SEATED OVERHEAD PRESS

The overhead press can be done seated or standing. It can also be done with a resistance band or dumbbells.

INSTRUCTIONS

1. Begin with arms out to the sides, with elbows bent at 90 degrees and palms facing forward.

2. Tighten your abdominals and avoid arching your back.

3. Press the dumbbells up and stop once your upper arms are fully extended. Do not lock out the elbows.

4. Lower to the starting position and begin again.

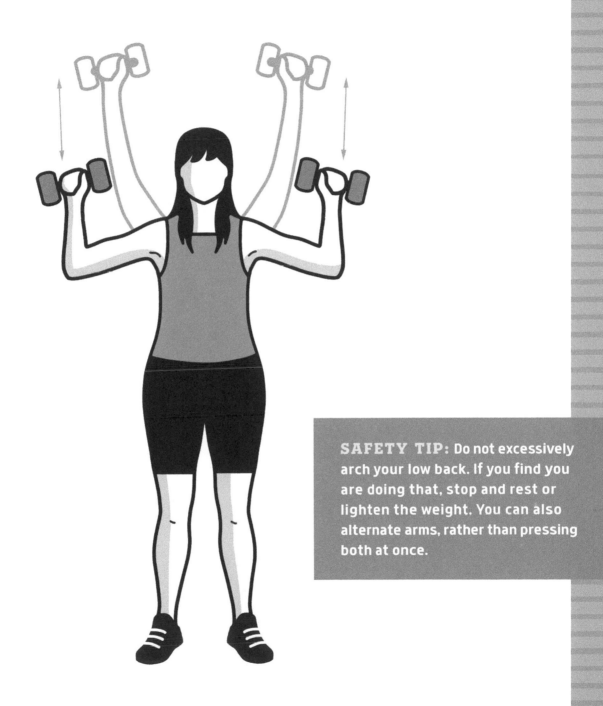

SAFETY TIP: Do not excessively arch your low back. If you find you are doing that, stop and rest or lighten the weight. You can also alternate arms, rather than pressing both at once.

muscle groups

Triceps

SINGLE-ARM TRICEPS KICKBACK

This exercise can be done with either a dumbbell or resistance band.

INSTRUCTIONS

1. Stand in a split stance, leaning forward to approximately 45 degrees.

2. Hold a dumbbell in one hand with the other hand on your leg, or support yourself by holding on to a stable object while in that position.

3. Extend the forearm back until your arm is straight and parallel to the floor.

4. Squeeze the back of your upper arm at the top of the motion before lowering.

5. Repeat to the desired number of reps.

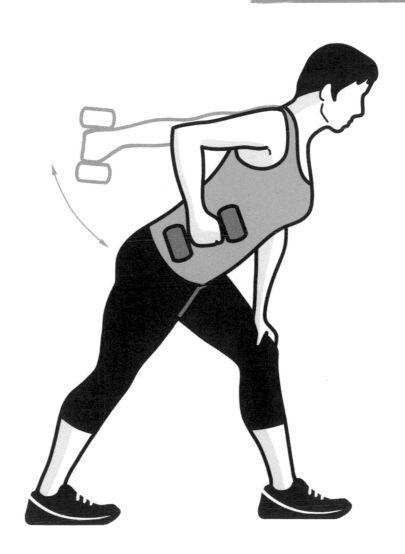

TIP: It's important to pause for a second or two while the arm is fully extended back so that you can squeeze the triceps. Use controlled motions in both directions.

muscle groups

Triceps

STANDING OVERHEAD TRICEPS EXTENSION

Strengthening the triceps will help you with functional strength, like pushing things away, pushing yourself up off the floor, or getting out of the tub.

INSTRUCTIONS

1. Start by standing with your feet shoulder-width apart and dumbbells held in front of you. Knees should be slightly bent.

2. Raise the dumbbells above your head until your arms are fully extended upward.

3. Slowly lower the weights back behind your head, being careful not to flare your elbows out too much.

4. Once your forearms dip below parallel to the floor, bring the weight back up to the starting position.

5. Squeeze your triceps at the top for a second or two before lowering again. Use slow, controlled motions.

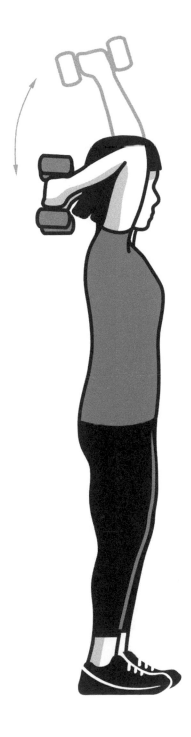

muscle groups

Biceps

Deltoids

Pectoralis Major

Pectoralis Minor

Trapezius

Triceps

BICEP CURL TO SHOULDER PRESS

Incorporating bicep curl and overhead press into one exercise allows you to quickly target many of the muscles in the upper body.

INSTRUCTIONS

1. Stand with your feet hip-distance apart. Hold one dumbbell in each hand next to your legs.

2. Bend your elbows and raise the dumbbells to your shoulders with your palms facing your chest.

3. Twist your hands so that your palms are facing away from you and push the dumbbells over your head.

4. Bend your elbows and lower the weights to your shoulders, twisting your wrists as you lower, so that your palms are again facing you.

5. Lower the weights to your sides into the starting position so that your palms are facing away from you at the bottom. Repeat to the desired number of reps.

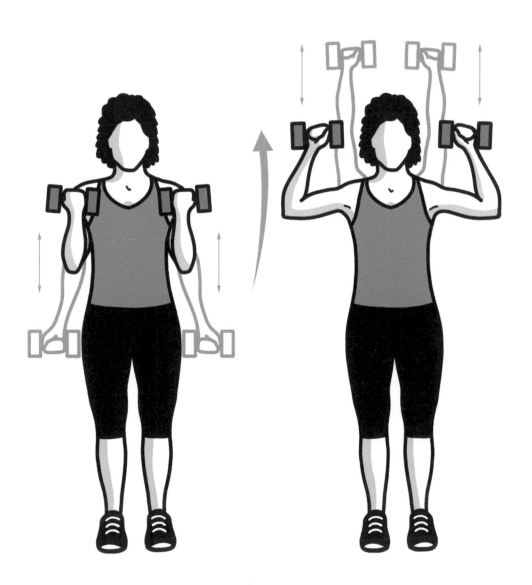

DUMBBELL (FREE WEIGHT) EXERCISES

muscle groups

Biceps

STANDING BICEP CURL WITH DUMBBELLS OR SMALL BARBELL

Standing bicep curls can also be done with a resistance band by standing in the middle of the band and holding the two handles as if they were dumbbells.

INSTRUCTIONS

1. Stand with your feet hip-distance apart and knees slightly bent.

2. Hold a dumbbell in each hand (or small barbell in both hands) slightly in front of your hips, with your palms facing forward. Lock your elbows into your sides.

3. Lift both dumbbells toward the shoulder until your palms are facing your shoulders and the elbow is pointing to the ground, with the forearm almost vertical.

4. Slowly lower the weight until your arms are fully or almost fully extended.

5. Repeat to the desired number of reps.

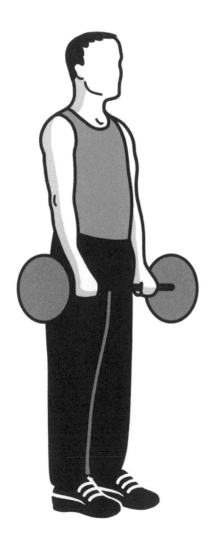

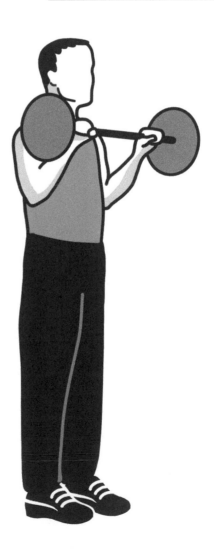

DUMBBELL (FREE WEIGHT) EXERCISES

muscle groups

Biceps

SEATED ALTERNATING BICEP CURL

Being seated and alternating arms both serve to make this version easier than standing and using both arms at once.

INSTRUCTIONS

1. At home, use a chair that gives enough clearance for your arms and dumbbells as you lower them. At the gym, sit at the end of a weight bench.

2. Begin with both arms relaxed and extended downward.

3. Lift one dumbbell toward your shoulder and slowly lower.

4. Once that dumbbell has been completely lowered, lift the other side. Completely lower the dumbbell and repeat on the original side.

5. Complete the desired number of reps on each side.

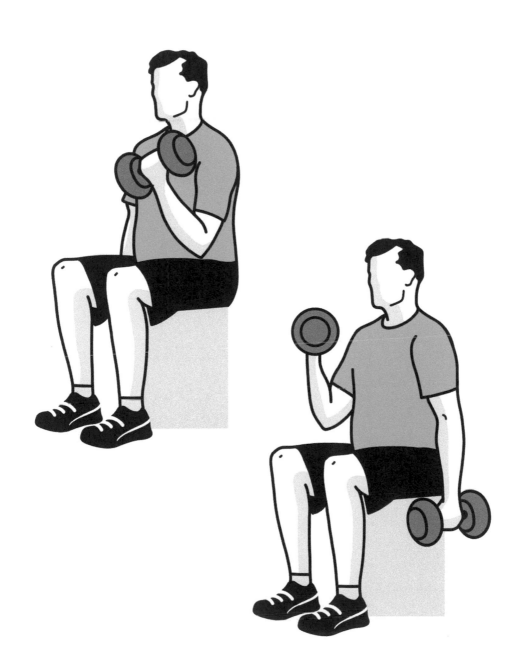

DUMBBELL (FREE WEIGHT) EXERCISES

muscle groups

Gastrocnemius

Soleus

DUMBBELL CALF RAISES

The calf muscles are often referred to as the second heart. So, you will want to keep those calves strong to help with blood circulation.

INSTRUCTIONS

1. Sit on a chair or bench with your feet flat on the floor and dumbbells positioned on your thighs but close to your knees.

2. Keeping the dumbbells firmly pressed against your knees, slowly raise your heels up off of the floor as far as possible, squeezing your calves and holding for a second or two.

3. Return back to the starting position and repeat to the desired number of reps.

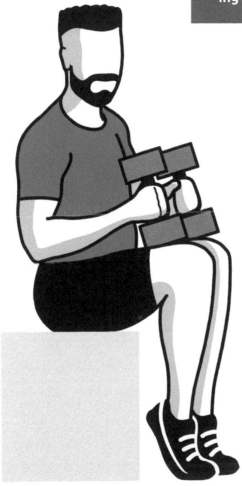

DUMBBELL (FREE WEIGHT) EXERCISES

muscle groups

Gastrocnemius

Glutes

Quadriceps

Soleus

SQUAT TO CALF RAISE

This is a variation on squats that guarantees to help with power, strength, and balance.

INSTRUCTIONS

1. Hold two dumbbells and stand with your feet hip-width apart and toes turned slightly outward.

2. Drop into a squat by hinging at your hips.

3. Drop your hips enough so that your thighs are parallel to the floor or below.

4. Once your legs are straight, lift your heels off of the ground and perform a calf raise onto the balls of your feet. Squeeze and hold for a second or two.

5. Drop your heels back down, returning to the bottom of the squat position.

6. Repeat to the desired number of reps.

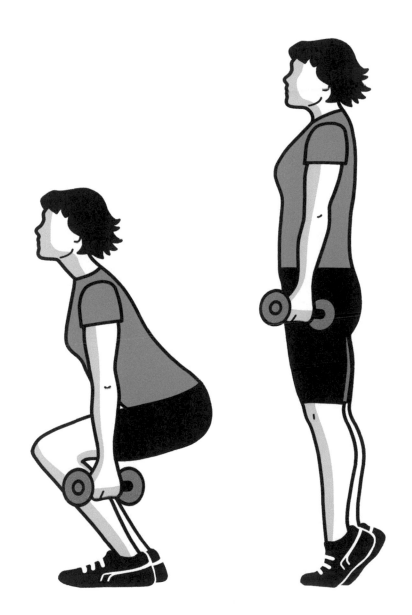

DUMBBELL (FREE WEIGHT) EXERCISES

muscle groups

Glutes

Quadriceps

DUMBBELL SQUATS

Once you have mastered the bodyweight squat, you can add resistance. You can do this either with the resistance band (page 126) or with dumbbells.

INSTRUCTIONS

1. Set your feet shoulder-width apart, toes slightly turned out.

2. Initiate the movement by pushing your hips back first. (Like you're shutting the car door with your glutes because your hands are full.)

3. Slowly bend at the knees, continuing to push your hips back until your thighs are as close to parallel to the floor as possible.

4. At the bottom of the movement, pause for a second or two and strongly push back up to the starting position.

5. Keep your chin parallel to the floor and keep your back straight.

6. Repeat to the desired number of reps.

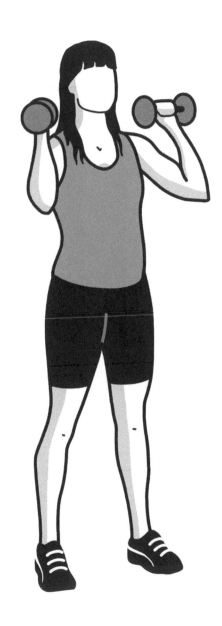
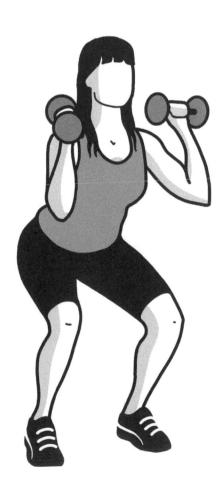

DUMBBELL (FREE WEIGHT) EXERCISES

muscle groups

> Glutes

> Hamstrings

SINGLE-LEG DEADLIFT

This is a great exercise for balance in addition to posterior-chain strength.

INSTRUCTIONS

1. Hold two dumbbells in front of your thighs, with your palms facing inward. If you need a little help with balance, stand alongside a wall or secure piece of gym equipment to use as a stabilizer when you feel wobbly. In this case, hold the dumbbell in the right hand and stand on the right leg with the wall to your left.

2. Slowly lift one leg straight behind you, bending the standing leg only slightly.

3. Hinge forward so that your arms lower the dumbbell(s) toward the floor. Keep your back flat.

4. You should feel a stretch in the standing-leg hamstring. Pause, then return to upright position.

5. Repeat to the desired number of reps before switching legs. *If using one dumbbell, turn around and work the opposite leg, with the wall on your other side.*

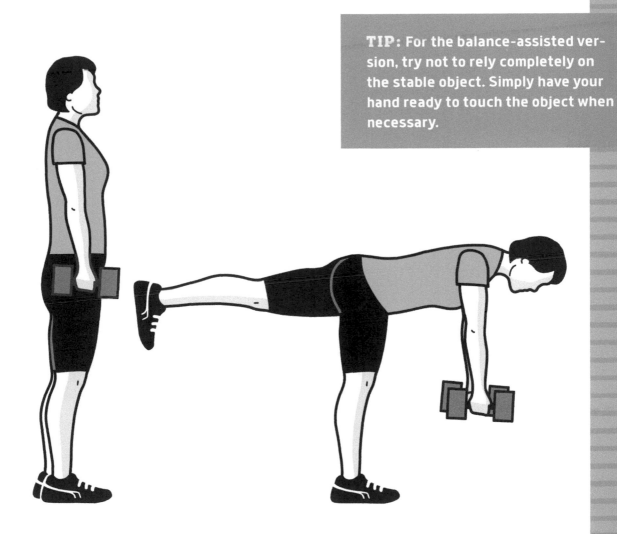

TIP: For the balance-assisted version, try not to rely completely on the stable object. Simply have your hand ready to touch the object when necessary.

DUMBBELL (FREE WEIGHT) EXERCISES

muscle groups

Glutes

Hamstrings

Quadriceps

Vastus Medialis

WALKING LUNGES

All the muscles utilized in this movement are important for everyday function and mobility.

INSTRUCTIONS

1. Find a location at home or in the gym where you can complete numerous steps in succession.

2. Begin by standing with your shoulders back and a dumbbell in each hand, hanging down at your sides. (Try without dumbbells at first if added weight is too challenging.)

3. Step forward with one leg, flexing the knees to drop straight down.

4. Descend until your rear knee nearly touches the ground and your front thigh is as close to parallel to the floor as possible.

5. Your posture should remain upright, and your front knee should stay above the front ankle.

6. Repeat to the desired number of reps with each leg.

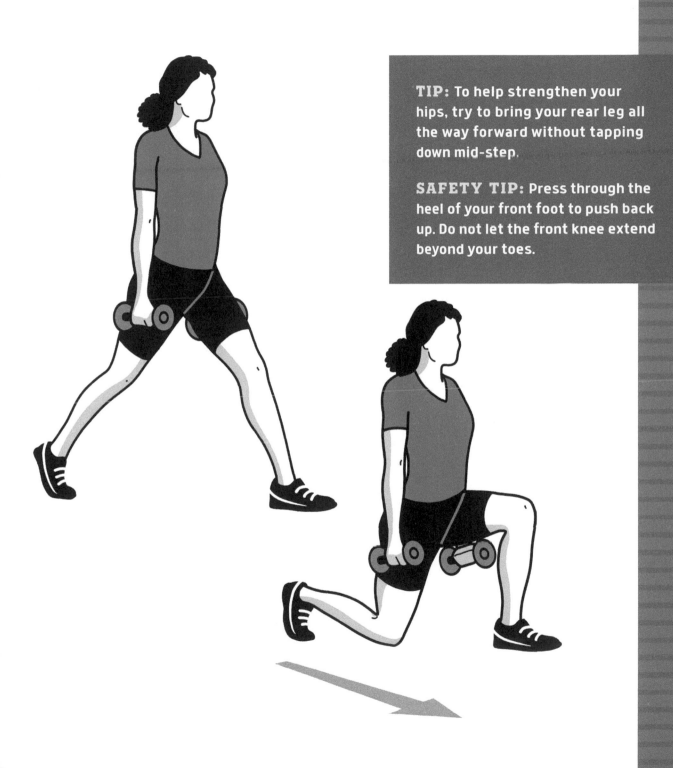

TIP: To help strengthen your hips, try to bring your rear leg all the way forward without tapping down mid-step.

SAFETY TIP: Press through the heel of your front foot to push back up. Do not let the front knee extend beyond your toes.

muscle groups

Biceps

Glutes

Quadriceps

SPLIT SQUAT WITH BICEP CURL

You can combine two exercises into one move to efficiently target even more muscles.

INSTRUCTIONS

1. Start in a split-stance position, with one leg forward and one leg back, with the rear heel off the floor.

2. Flex your knees and drop straight down until the back knee is just above the floor. Squeeze your biceps and curl the dumbbells upward.

3. Stand back up by pushing through the front heel, and slowly lower the arms. Keep your shoulders back and body upright.

4. Return to the starting position and repeat to the desired number of reps. Switch legs and repeat.

SAFETY TIP: Tuck your elbows into your torso throughout the movement to avoid swinging the dumbbells and rocking your torso.

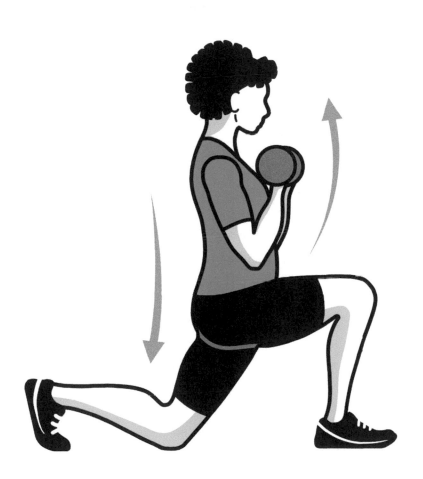

DUMBBELL (FREE WEIGHT) EXERCISES

muscle groups

Biceps

Glutes

Quadriceps

REVERSE LUNGE WITH BICEP CURL

Reverse lunges put less stress on your knees than the forward lunge and give you a bit more stability in your front leg.

INSTRUCTIONS

1. Start by standing with your feet shoulder-width apart, holding a dumbbell in each hand by your side.

2. Step back (about two feet) with your left foot, landing on the ball of your left foot and keeping your heel off the ground.

3. Bend both knees to create two 90-degree angles with your legs while lifting the dumbbells upwards, bringing palms towards your chest. Keep elbows tucked into your torso.

4. In this positioning, your shoulders should be directly above your hips and your chest should be upright (no leaning forward or back). Your right shin should be perpendicular to the floor and your right knee should be stacked above your right ankle. Your glutes and core should be engaged.

5. Push through the heel of your right foot to return to standing.

6. Repeat to the desired number of reps on each side.

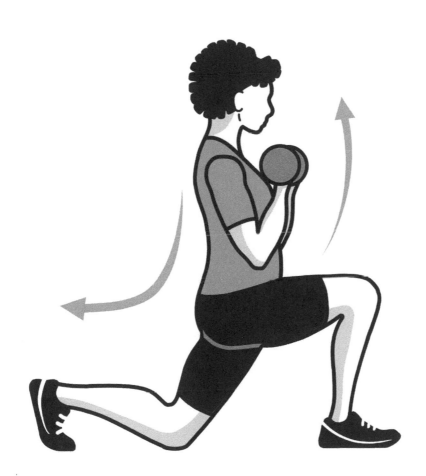

muscle groups

Abdominals ▶

Deltoids ▶

Glutes ▶

Quadriceps ▶

SQUATS WITH OVERHEAD PRESS

This exercise begins with a squat and ends with an overhead press and works the entire body in a single fluid motion. It helps improve coordination, muscular endurance, and balance. It also develops core stability.

INSTRUCTIONS

1. Stand tall with your back and legs straight, feet hip-distance apart, and toes pointing forward. Hold the dumbbells in front of your shoulders, with elbows bent and your palms facing outward.

2. Bend your knees and hips to squat down, keeping the chest lifted, back straight, and knees behind your toes.

3. Straighten your legs to the starting position.

4. Press the weights overhead in line with your shoulders to straighten (but not lock) the arms, with your palms facing outward.

5. Slowly lower the weights back down in front of your shoulders to complete one rep.

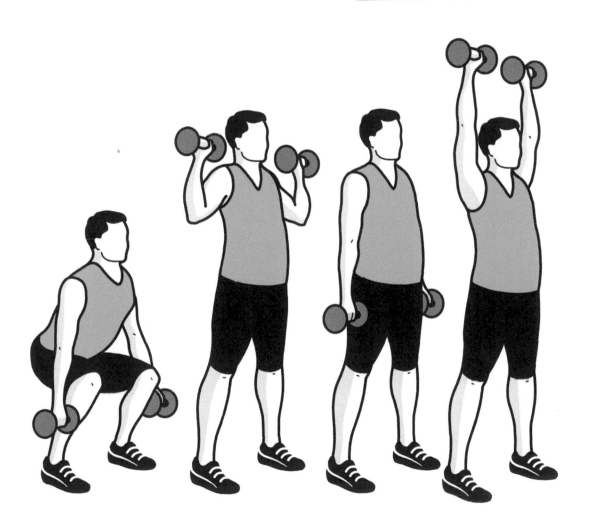

muscle groups

Adductors

Glutes

Shoulders

SUMO SQUAT WITH FRONT SHOULDER RAISE

Glute activation in the squat phase of the exercise makes it a fantastic exercise for lower body strength, while the front raise will help improve shoulder strength and mobility.

INSTRUCTIONS

1. Stand with your feet wider than shoulder-width apart and your toes turned out.

2. Hold a dumbbell in each hand in front of your hips.

3. Push your hips back and squat down, keeping your chest up and knees out.

4. As you squat down, lower the dumbbells in a slow, controlled manner, so that they are between your knees at the bottom of the movement.

5. Return to a standing position while extending your arms straight out in front of you until they're parallel to the floor.

6. Repeat to the desired number of reps.

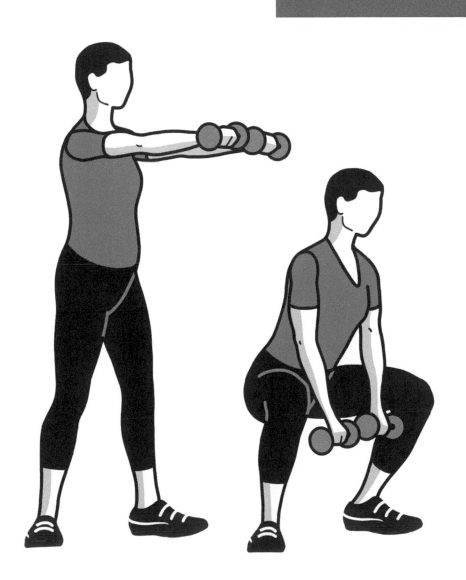

muscle groups

Adductors

Biceps

Glutes

Hamstrings

Quadriceps

LATERAL LUNGE WITH BICEP CURL

Increasing lateral stability is key for injury prevention and enhanced performance with everyday life.

INSTRUCTIONS

1. Start with your feet hip-width apart and dumbbells in hand.

2. Take a large step and lunge out to the right. Concentrate on sitting back into the right hip. Keep your torso as upright as possible.

3. With your palms facing upward, curl your arms up toward your shoulders, contracting your biceps as you step. Keep your elbows close to your sides.

4. Push off the bent leg and return back to standing. Alternate legs.

5. Repeat to the desired number of reps on each side.

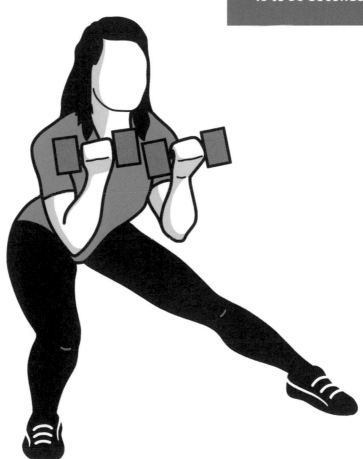

RESISTANCE BAND & STABILITY BALL EXERCISES

Having resistance bands at home will increase your strength training options and are a perfect progression from simple bodyweight exercises. They are inexpensive and come in a variety of strengths. They are also perfect for traveling! A stability ball also adds to home workout options and are typically available in all gyms.

muscle groups

Latissimus Dorsi

Trapezius

Rhomboids

Rear Deltoids

SEATED ROW (ON FLOOR)

The seated cable row is a pulling exercise that is great for the back, shoulders, and arms.

INSTRUCTIONS

1. Sit down on the floor with your chest up, back flat, and legs extended in front of you.

2. Wrap the resistance band around the bottom of your feet.

3. Hold the handles (if you have the kind with handles) or the ends of a continuous-loop resistance band with your hands, using a neutral, palms-facing-in grip with your arms extended in front of you.

4. Pull toward your torso, squeezing your shoulder blades as you pull.

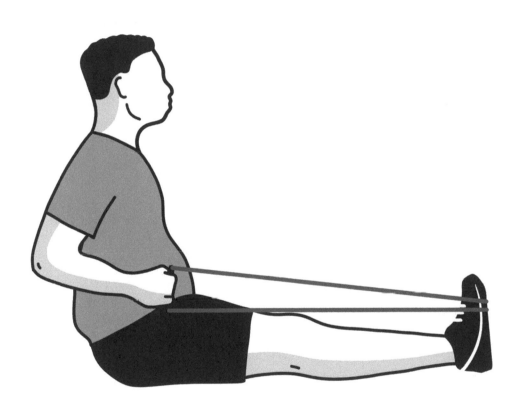

SAFETY TIP: Keep your upper body stationary. Do not use momentum as you pull and release.

muscle groups

Trapezius

Rear Deltoids

Rhomboids

PULL-APARTS

The band pull-apart is an essential exercise for those who spend most of their day hunched over a computer keyboard.

INSTRUCTIONS

1. Start with a band of appropriate tension.

2. Keep your arms, elbows, and wrists straight and fully extended in front of you.

3. With your arms parallel to the floor and your palms facing down, slowly pull the band apart while keeping your arms straight.

4. Pull until your arms are directly out to your sides, straight, and parallel to the floor.

5. Squeeze your shoulder blades together while keeping your shoulders down.

6. Hold the fully contracted position for two seconds, then return to the starting position.

7. Repeat to complete 12 repetitions, using slow, controlled motions.

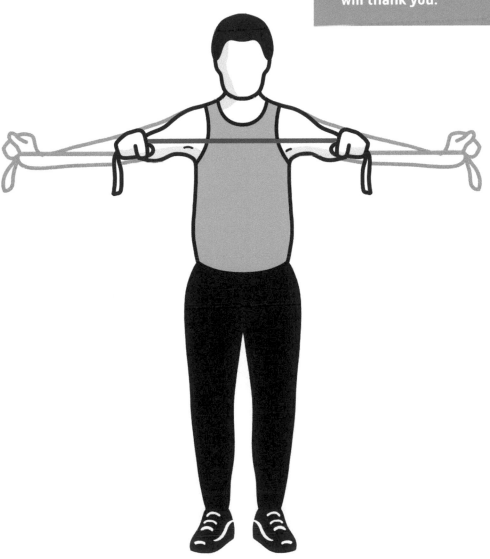

TIP: Having a resistance band on hand at the office is a great idea. Take a few minutes every hour or two to do this exercise. Your body will thank you.

muscle groups

> **Medial Deltoid**

LATERAL SHOULDER RAISE

The lateral raise is an upper body isolation exercise for building shoulder strength. This exercise can be done with dumbbells or a resistance band.

INSTRUCTIONS

1. Stand on the exact middle of the band while holding the ends in each hand.

2. Begin with your arms by your sides with your palms facing inward.

3. Adjust the amount of play you have with the band by standing on it with one foot or both feet. Keeping your arms straight, slowly raise your arms to the sides until shoulder height and parallel to the floor.

4. Slowly return to the starting position and repeat with slow, controlled motions.

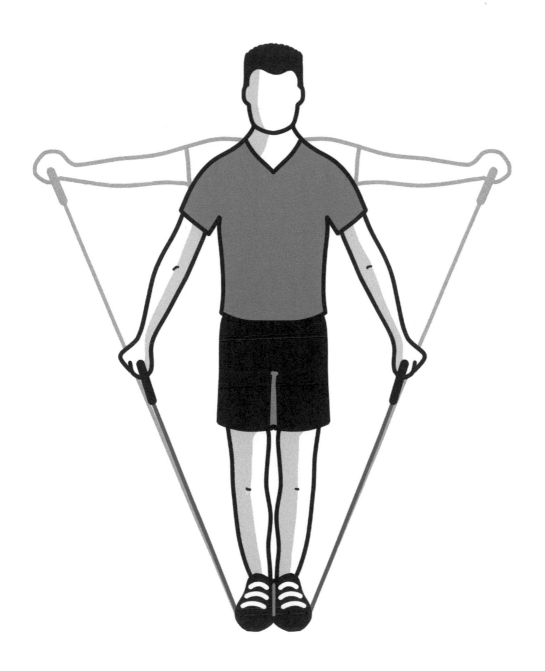

muscle groups

Pectoralis Major

Pectoralis Minor

Triceps

LYING CHEST PRESS (FLOOR)

This is an amazing at-home option for the popular bench press.

INSTRUCTIONS

1. Adjust the grip position on the band so that you have the appropriate tension as you extend your arms. You *need* to feel resistance as you push. (The less band you have to work with, the more challenging the exercise will be.)

2. Extend both arms until they're straight, pulling the band up with them.

3. Keep your spine flat throughout the exercise. Lower your arms back to the starting position and repeat.

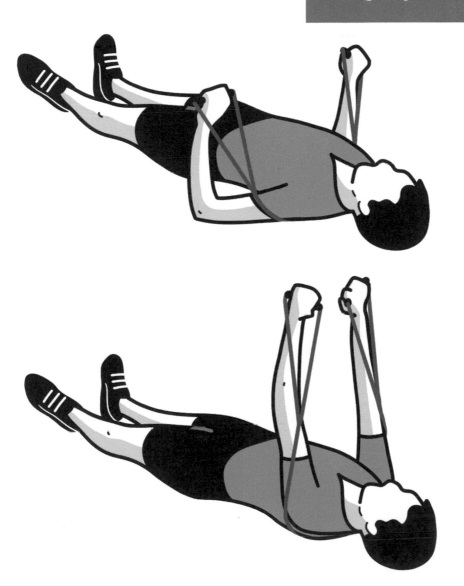

TIP: You can also do this movement in the standing position by wrapping the band around a sturdy pole and facing away from the anchor point.

muscle groups

Biceps

Latissimus Dorsi

Rhomboids

BENT-OVER ROW

Bent-over rows are most often performed with dumbbells or a barbell, but this important exercise can also be done with resistance bands.

INSTRUCTIONS

1. Begin the movement by stepping onto a resistance band with your feet at shoulder width and your toes pointed slightly out.

2. Bend slightly at the knees and forward at the hips. Maintain a braced core and flat back throughout.

3. Leading with your elbows, pull the handles of the resistance band back, bringing your shoulder blades closer together. Hold this contraction and slowly release to the starting position.

4. Be sure you don't have too much slack in the band in the bottom of the movement. You want to maintain slight tension throughout.

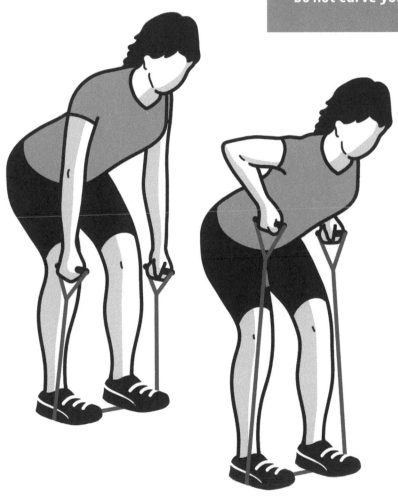

TIP: If you have too much slack in the band, adjust your grip farther down the band, or gather it up between your feet.

SAFETY TIP: Keep your back flat. Do not curve your spine forward.

muscle groups

Deltoids

Pectoralis Major

Pectoralis Minor

Trapezius

Triceps

OVERHEAD PRESS

The overhead press is a compound movement that builds strong shoulders, chest, and arms while also working your core muscles.

INSTRUCTIONS

1. Place both feet in the exact middle of the resistance band.

2. Tighten your abdominals and avoid arching your back.

3. Press the handles of the resistance band up and stop once your upper arms are fully extended. The band should be behind your arms.

4. Slowly press the resistance band overhead. Do not lock out the elbows. Lower to the starting position and begin again.

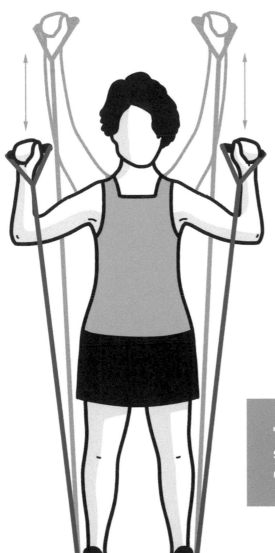

TIP: If there is too much tension, stand in a split stance with only one foot in the center of the band.

muscle groups

Triceps

BENT-OVER TRICEPS EXTENSION

The triceps help stabilize your shoulder joint and extend the arm at the shoulder and elbow.

INSTRUCTIONS

1. Holding one end of the band in each hand, stand in the center of the band with your feet shoulder-width apart.

2. Bend forward at your hips to approximately, but no more than, 90 degrees, so that your back is as close to parallel to the ground as possible.

3. Hold the band with your palms facing inward.

4. Bend your elbows so that they are tight against your ribs.

5. As you exhale, extend your arms behind you until they're fully extended and parallel to the floor.

6. Inhale as you bend your elbows again.

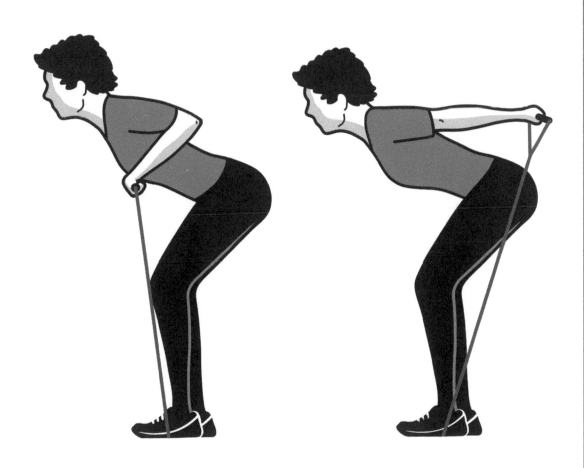

muscle groups

Adductors

Glutes

Quadriceps

SUMO (OR REGULAR STANCE) SQUATS WITH STABILITY BALL (BODYWEIGHT OR DUMBBELLS)

This is a great exercise option if you feel a little unsteady on your feet while squatting.

INSTRUCTIONS

1. Position the stability ball in the small of your back with the ball against an unobstructed wall.

2. Place your feet out in front of you, either in a sumo stance (feet pointed outward) or straight ahead. Your feet should be far enough out front so that your knees are bent at 90 degrees when in the lower position.

3. Squat down until your thighs are parallel to the floor or as close as you can come to that position.

4. Whether using bodyweight or dumbbells, the movement is the same. Use slow, fluid motion, and push up through your heels.

5. Repeat to the desired number of reps.

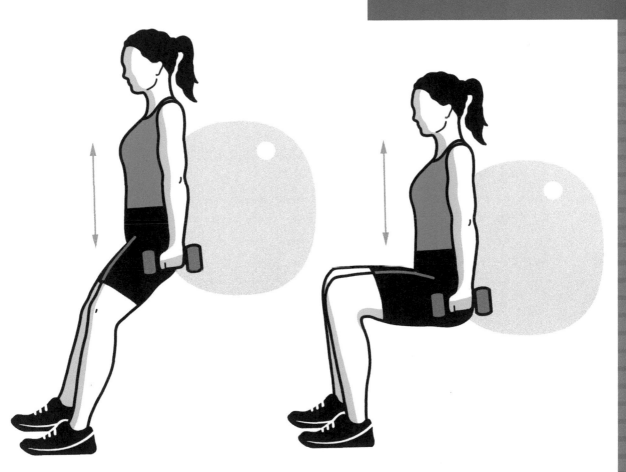

TIP: If you are using dumbbells be sure to have placed them on the floor where you can pick them up when you're in the squat position. Set them down again when you're done with your reps.

muscle groups

Glutes

Quadriceps

SQUATS WITH RESISTANCE BAND

The band adds resistance to the bodyweight version of this exercise in the same way that holding two dumbbells does.

INSTRUCTIONS

1. Stand on the band with your feet shoulder-width apart.

2. Hold the handles next to your shoulders so the band is behind the back of your arms.

3. Slowly sit back into the squat position, keeping your abdominals tight and chest lifted.

4. Lower until your thighs are parallel to the floor or as close to parallel as you can come.

5. Press back up through the heels to a standing position, squeezing the glutes at the top as you tuck your hips under your ribcage.

6. Repeat to the desired number of reps.

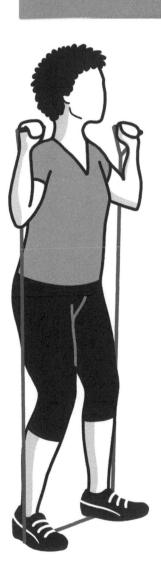

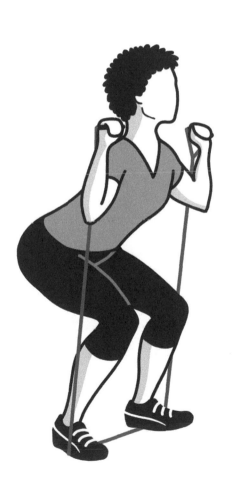

TIP: If you need to add more resistance, either gather some band between your feet, or wrap the band around your hands a time or two, to take up some slack.

RESISTANCE BAND & STABILITY BALL EXERCISES

muscle groups

Abdominal

Hamstrings

HAMSTRING ROLL-IN WITH STABILITY BALL

This is a simple but effective exercise to strengthen your hamstrings, glutes, and core muscles.

INSTRUCTIONS

1. Lie on the floor with your arms at your sides and place your heels on the ball. Press up so that your hips are in the air and your torso forms a straight line.

2. Next, pull the ball toward you, squeezing your hamstrings.

3. Roll the ball back out without dropping your hips. It's imperative that you keep your hips raised throughout the movement.

TIP: You can make this more challenging by placing your hands on your belly so that you can't brace yourself with your arms on the floor.

muscle groups

> Glutes

> Hamstrings

ROMANIAN DEADLIFT WITH BAND OR DUMBBELLS

The Romanian deadlift is an exercise that works the posterior chain of muscles that run down the back of our bodies and are responsible for our upright posture.

INSTRUCTIONS

1. If using a band, step on the center of a continuous loop or a handled resistance band.

2. Bend over while holding the end loops or the handles. If using dumbbells, hinge forward at the hips, keeping your back flat, holding a dumbbell in each hand with your palms facing your legs.

3. If using the band, gather as much of it as necessary to increase the resistance. Or simply hold the band farther down so that there is very little "play" in the band. (You will find the spot to hold that creates the resistance that you need to complete your reps with the appropriate amount of tension.)

4. With your hips pushed back and back flat, stand straight while holding the band ends or dumbbells.

5. Slowly lower again by pushing your hips back and keeping your back flat until you feel the stretch in the backs of your legs (hamstrings).

6. Only slightly bend your knees as you bend forward.

7. Repeat to the desired number of reps.

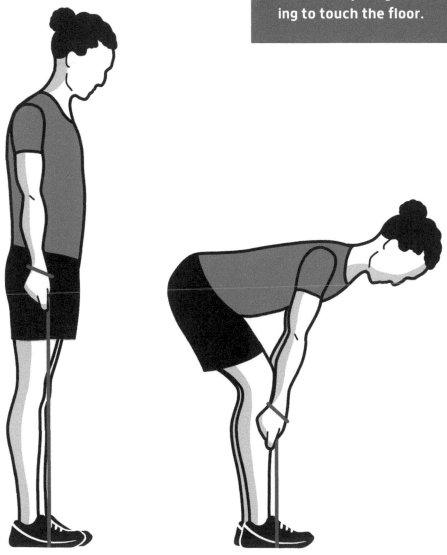

SAFETY TIP: Do not round your back. There is no movement other than the hip hinge. You are not trying to touch the floor.

GYM MACHINE EXERCISES

Most gym machines will have instructions written on them. If the instructions are unclear, do not hesitate to ask the gym staff for assistance. They are there to help you. Using machines is a safe place to begin strength training at the gym.

muscle groups

Pectoralis Major

Triceps

CHEST PRESS (FIXED RESISTANCE)

This machine mimics a push-up or bench press. It is a safe option for strengthening your chest and triceps, especially if you've never strength trained before.

INSTRUCTIONS

1. Have a seat and grasp the handles.

2. Push the handles straight out in front, until your arms are fully extended but not locked.

3. Slowly return to the starting position, being mindful of not letting your arms drift past your shoulder.

4. Repeat to the desired number of reps.

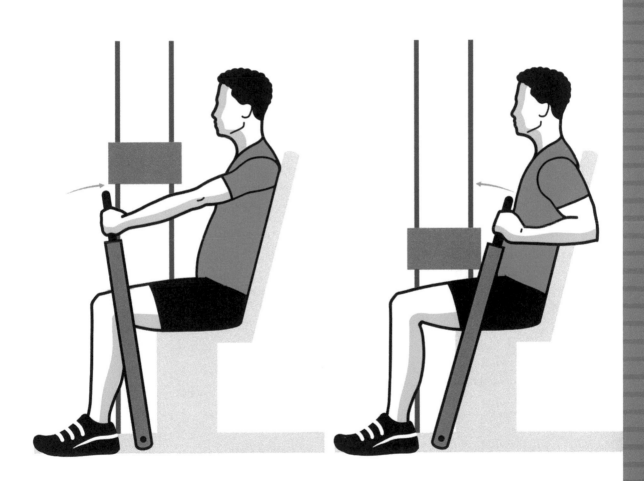

muscle groups

Biceps

Latissimus Dorsi

LAT PULL-DOWN

It is a challenge to replicate this movement at home unless you can do a pull-up, which most people cannot do.

INSTRUCTIONS

1. Adjust the pad so it sits snugly on your thighs to minimize using momentum.

2. Grasp the bar with a wide grip, looking forward with your torso upright. (If you're short like I am, you will have to grab the bar while standing and sit down with it held above your head.)

3. Focus on squeezing your shoulder blades together as you pull the bar down in front of you to your upper chest. Resist the temptation to lean back to aid the movement.

4. Keep your arms out to the sides as you pull down, leading with your elbows. Do not allow arms to drift forward as you fatigue.

5. Slowly return to the top position and repeat with slow, controlled motions until you've reached the desired number of reps.

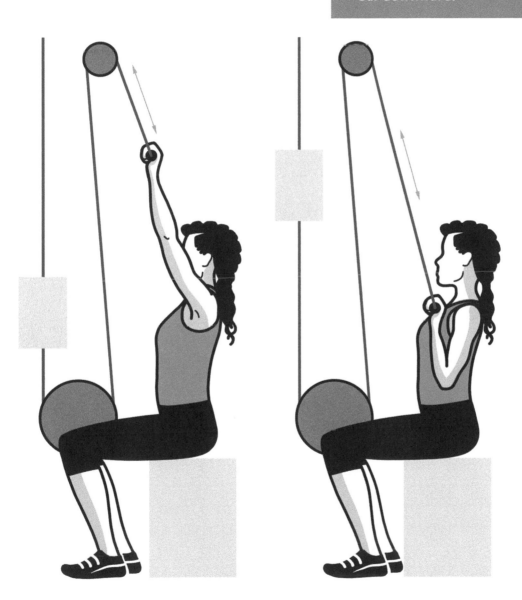

TIP: Resist the temptation to use momentum, by rocking back and forth, to aid in pulling the bar downward.

muscle groups

Latissimus Dorsi

Rear Deltoids

Trapezius

Rhomboids

SEATED CABLE ROW

The seated cable row develops the muscles of the back and the forearms, and is a staple among gym-goers.

INSTRUCTIONS

1. Position yourself on the seat with your knees slightly bent so that you can reach the handle with outstretched arms. Keep your back flat.

2. Pull the handle and weight toward the lower abdomen while trying not to use the momentum by moving the torso backward and forward. Squeeze your shoulder blades together as you row, keeping your chest up.

3. Return the handle forward under tension to full stretch, remembering to keep that back flat even though flexed at the hips.

4. Repeat to the desired number of reps.

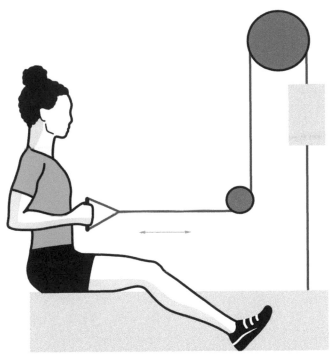

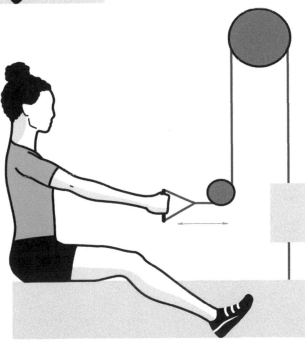

muscle groups

Latissimus Dorsi

Rear Deltoids

Rhomboids

Trapezius

SEATED ROW (FIXED RESISTANCE)

This machine is an alternative to the cable row and the dumbbell and resistance band rows.

INSTRUCTIONS

1. Make any necessary adjustments to the seat or chest pad. (Most machines usually have guidelines for height adjustments as well as instructions.)

2. Grip the handles by reaching in front of you. You may have the option of a vertical or horizontal handle. Use the one that feels the most comfortable to you.

3. Pull the handles, bending your elbows and pointing them out to the sides, as you focus on squeezing your shoulder blades together.

4. Slowly straighten the arms to the starting position to complete one rep.

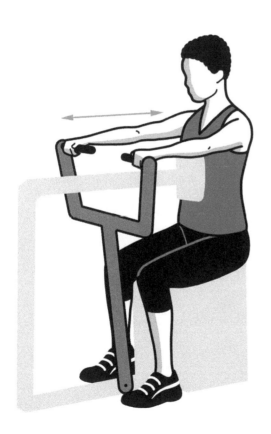

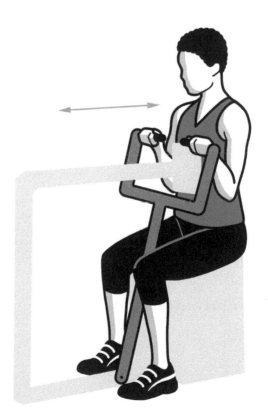

muscle groups

Glutes

Quadriceps

LEG PRESS MACHINE

Leg press machines are an awesome place to start for people who haven't exercised in a while or who are rehabilitating from a joint surgery or injury because there is little chance of losing proper form.

INSTRUCTIONS

1. Sit yourself down on the machine and experiment with the weight by starting light and finding the weight that fatigues the muscles in the 10 to 15 rep range. Your knees should be as close to 90 degrees as possible.

2. If it is the type of machine where you have to add weight plates, press without any added weights at first. There is always some resistance to the machines even without weight, especially with the vertical style.

3. Press so that your legs are fully extended, but do not lock your knees.

4. Push through your heels.

5. Slowly return until your knees are back to 90 degrees and repeat, using slow, controlled motions.

6. Repeat to the desired number of reps.

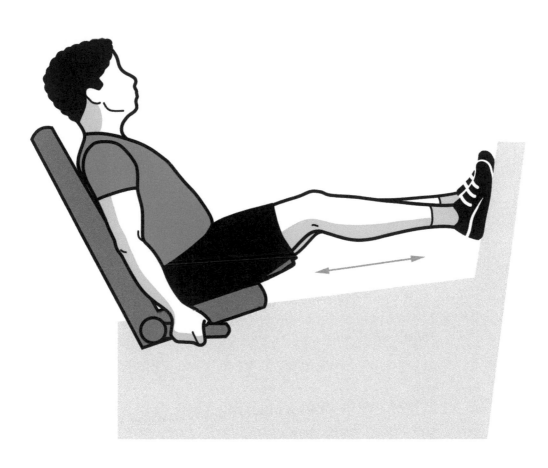

muscle groups

Gastrocnemius

Soleus

CALF RAISES ON LEG PRESS

I often program the calf raises between leg press sets for my clients. If you are doing two sets of each exercise, you will do the leg press, calf raise, leg press, calf raise. This is called super-setting.

INSTRUCTIONS

1. Once you have completed a set of leg presses, fully extend your legs and walk your feet down to the bottom of the plate so that the balls of your feet are on the bottom edge of the foot plate, with toes facing upward. (You will not have to change the weight.)

2. Press upward as if you are standing on your tiptoes. Squeeze your calf muscles as you press.

3. Slowly, lower your heels below the foot plate if possible, for greater range of motion. (People with plantar fasciitis find this stretch feels particularly good.)

4. Press back up onto the balls of your feet and repeat to desired number of reps.

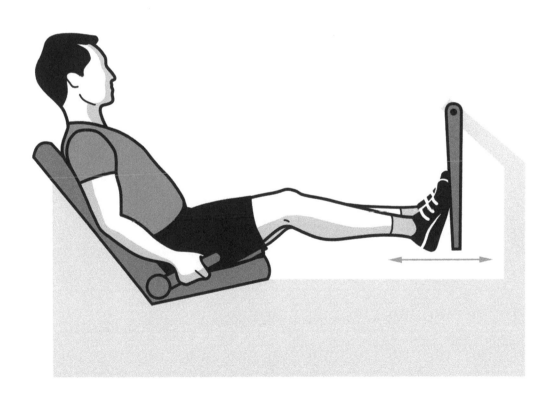

TIP: You can target the calf muscles differently by changing the position of your feet. If you want to target the inner calf, point the feet outward. Conversely, if you want to target the outer portion, point your toes slightly inward.

muscle groups

Hamstrings

HAMSTRING CURL MACHINE

There are different versions of the hamstring curl machine, and your gym will have at least one version of it. The seated model is shown here, but there are lying and standing versions as well.

INSTRUCTIONS

1. Sit in the leg curl machine and place your calves on top of the padded lever.

2. Lower the thigh support so that it rests just above your knees.

3. Holding the handles for support and keeping your back pressed into the seat, pull your heels all the way to the back of your thighs. Hold for a count of two, squeezing your hamstrings.

4. Slowly return to the starting position, with your legs fully extended in front of you.

5. Repeat to the desired number of reps.

TIP: Try to relax your lower legs so that your calf muscles don't try to take over for your hamstrings.

PART 2

Get
Stronger
THE 6-WEEK PROGRAM

Strength training may be *way* outside your comfort zone, but that's where the best things happen. Make a promise to yourself that you will follow through to the end of the six weeks and carry your newfound knowledge forward. Of course, you cannot get strong overnight, but if you stick with it, you *will* get a stronger, more functional body.

The most important weight training principle is this: Choose a weight that creates a *real effort* by the last couple of repetitions. You must *work* to get those last reps finished, or your body will not get stronger. Simply going through the motions will get you nowhere. However, we never want to sacrifice proper form for those last repetitions. If you find yourself using momentum or incorporating muscles other than the ones you're targeting, it's time to stop that set. It's important to use controlled motions in all phases of any exercise.

I suggest you keep a record of the weights you're using for each exercise. It will allow you to see the number increase over time and will give you an undeniable sense of accomplishment.

You'll notice that I've recommended doing two sets of each exercise for the first two weeks and increased to three sets from the third week onward. I've found that three sets of 10 to 12 reps is a well-rounded and sustainable way to train for almost everyone. However, if you find three sets is a little too much, stay with two sets until you feel that you are ready to add another.

I am truly excited for you and this path you've chosen. Strength training is one of the best things we can do for our health and for ourselves.

Inspiration for This Week

Believe in yourself and all that you are. Know that there is something inside of you that is greater than any obstacle.

–CHRISTIAN D. LARSON

chapter 4

Week 1

This week will lay the foundation for the weeks to come. We will be working out two to three days this week. Choose whether you will be working out at home or in a gym, and then follow the exercise program that pertains to your choice. If you dedicate yourself to each rep and set, I promise you will begin to grow stronger and you will feel the difference.

WEEK 1: HOME WORKOUT

Day of the Week: Choose two to three days for this week's workout, with a day of rest between workouts.

Approximate Workout Time: 35 minutes (including 5-minute warm-up and 10-minute cooldown)

Overview: These should be bodyweight exercises. No equipment is needed until week 2. Two sets of 12 repetitions (both sides) with 1-minute rest between sets.

Reminder: Warm-up, page 22; Cooldown, pages 22 to 41

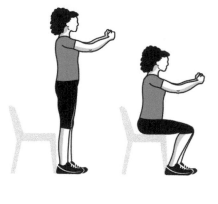

BODYWEIGHT CHAIR SQUATS
PAGE 60

OR (more challenging)

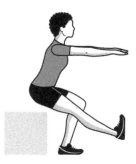

SINGLE-LEG SQUAT TO CHAIR
PAGE 62

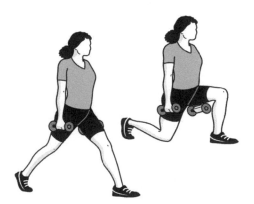

**SPLIT SQUATS
(WITH BODYWEIGHT
OR DUMBBELLS)**
PAGE 64

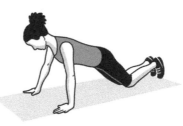

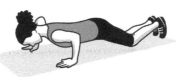

PUSH-UP FROM KNEES
PAGE 52

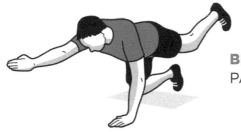

BIRD DOG
PAGE 58

**TRICEPS DIP FROM
CHAIR WITH BENT LEGS**
PAGE 56

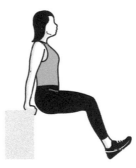

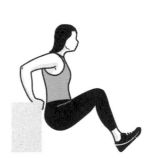

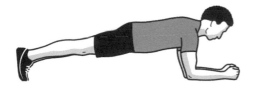

15-SECOND FOREARM PLANK
PAGE 42

WEEK 1: GYM WORKOUT

Day of the Week: Choose two to three days for this week's workout with a day of rest between workouts.

Approximate Workout Time: 35 minutes (including 5-minute warm-up and 10-minute cooldown)

Overview: Two sets of 12 reps (both sides). One-minute rest between sets.

Reminder: Warm-up, page 22; Cooldown, pages 22 to 41

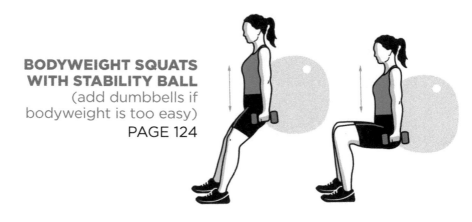

BODYWEIGHT SQUATS WITH STABILITY BALL
(add dumbbells if bodyweight is too easy)
PAGE 124

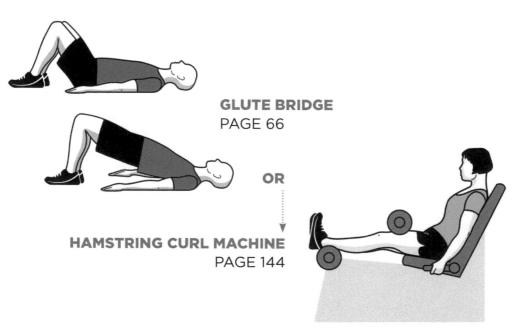

GLUTE BRIDGE
PAGE 66

OR

HAMSTRING CURL MACHINE
PAGE 144

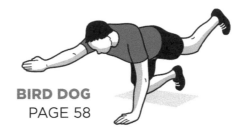

BIRD DOG
PAGE 58

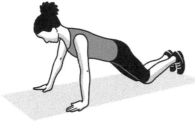

PUSH-UP FROM KNEES
PAGE 52

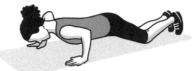

OR

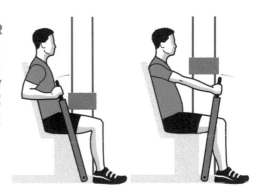

CHEST PRESS MACHINE
PAGE 132

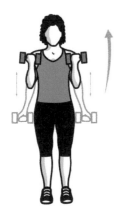

**STANDING BICEP CURL
WITH DUMBBELLS OR
SMALL BARBELL**
PAGE 86

**15- TO 30-SECOND
FOREARM PLANK**
PAGE 42

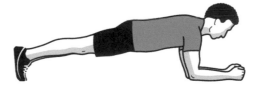

SELF CHECK-IN WORKSHEET

1. How motivated was I to complete the fitness program each day? Is there anything I could do differently to improve my motivation?

   » *Surround yourself with people who want you to succeed with your fitness goals.*

2. Did I notice any changes in appetite this week? (Was I hungrier/less hungry?)

   » *Did I crave any different foods than normal? Many people find that keeping a food journal helps keep them on track with nutrition.*

3. Did I make a conscious effort to drink more water?

   » *Many people find that carrying a water bottle will ensure that they get into the habit of drinking more water.*

4. Did I make an effort to get more sleep? Was my sleep of better, the same, or worse quality?

   » *Science shows that a bedtime routine will set you up for a better night's sleep.*

5. Did I find that some of the exercises were too challenging or too easy?

   » *If too challenging, do only as many repetitions as you comfortably can and build to 10 to 12 over time as you adapt. If too easy, add weight or do the more advanced version if one was given.*

Notes

Inspiration for This Week

Gratitude and attitude are not challenges; they are choices.

-ROBERT BRAATHE

chapter 5

Week 2

By this week you will need at least two to three dumbbells or two to three resistance bands of various strengths for your home workout. You can find resistance bands online or in your local sporting goods store.

It is difficult to advise as to the specific weight or strength of those dumbbells and bands, but in general, I suggest the following guidelines for men and women who have never lifted weights before:

For a woman under 55 years: 5 lb, 8 lb, and 12/15 lb dumbbells
For a man under 55 years: 8 lb, 10 lb, and 15/20 lb dumbbells
For a woman over 55 years: 3/5 lb, 8 lb, and 10 lb dumbbells
For a man over 55 years: 5 lb, 10 lb, and 12 lb dumbbells

WEEK 2: HOME WORKOUT

Day of the Week: Choose three days for this week's workout, with a day of rest between workouts.

Approximate Workout Time: 35 minutes (including 5-minute warm-up and 10-minute cooldown)

Overview: Bodyweight, dumbbells, and bands. Two sets of 12 repetitions (both sides) with 1 minute rest between sets.

Reminder: Warm-up, page 22; Cooldown, pages 22 to 41

BODYWEIGHT SQUATS
PAGE 60

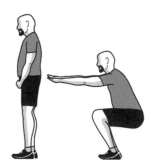

OR (more challenging)

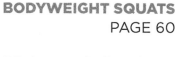

SQUATS WITH RESISTANCE BAND
PAGE 126

SPLIT SQUAT WITH BICEP CURL
PAGE 100

RESISTANCE BAND ROWS
PAGE 118

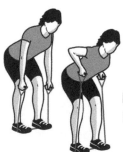

BENT-OVER ROW
PAGE 70

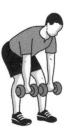
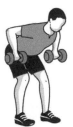

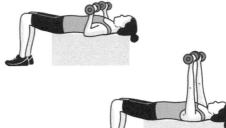

CHEST PRESS WITH DUMBBELLS
PAGE 72

OR

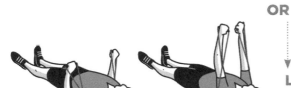

LYING BAND CHEST PRESS
PAGE 116

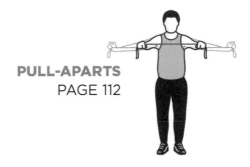

PULL-APARTS
PAGE 112

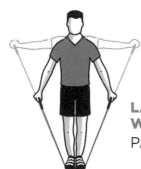

LATERAL SHOULDER RAISE WITH RESISTANCE BAND
PAGE 114

OR

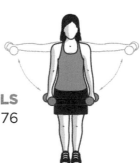

LATERAL RAISE WITH DUMBBELLS
PAGE 76

WEEK 2: GYM WORKOUT

Day of the Week: Choose three days for this week's workout, with a day of rest between workouts.

Approximate Workout Time: 35 minutes (including 5-minute warm-up and 10-minute cooldown)

Overview: Dumbbells and machines. Two sets of 12 repetitions (both sides) with 1 minute rest between sets.

Reminder: Warm-up, page 22; Cooldown, pages 22 to 41

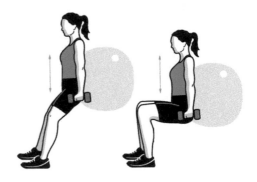

BODYWEIGHT SUMO SQUATS WITH STABILITY BALL

OR

DUMBBELL SUMO SQUATS WITH STABILITY BALL
PAGE 124

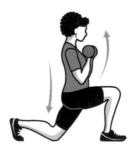

SPLIT SQUAT WITH BICEP CURL
PAGE 100

STANDING OR SEATED OVERHEAD PRESS
PAGE 78

LAT PULL-DOWN MACHINE
PAGE 134

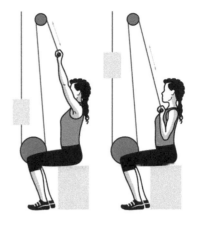

OR

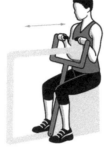
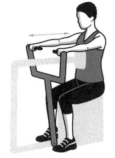

SEATED ROW ON FIXED MACHINE
PAGE 138

SEATED CABLE ROW
PAGE 136

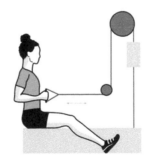
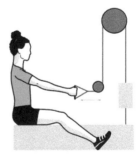
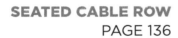

CHEST PRESS WITH DUMBBELLS
PAGE 72

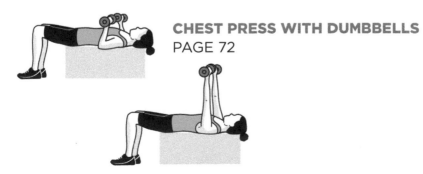

SELF CHECK-IN WORKSHEET

1. How motivated was I to exercise compared to last week? Was I looking forward to working out?

    » *Continue to surround yourself with people who want you to succeed with your fitness goals. Perhaps go back to the beginning of this book and remind yourself why it's so important to keep our bodies strong.*

2. Did I notice any changes in appetite this week? Did I find that I am more aware of what I'm eating?

    » *If you've started a food journal, try to keep it up to date. It's one of the best tools for making us more aware of what we are actually eating.*

3. Am I keeping on top of my water intake? If not, is there anything I can do to help me drink more water?

    » *Keeping water with you at all times may help. Some people like to flavor their water with lemon wedges or cucumber slices.*

4. How is my energy level? Am I getting enough sleep? Has my energy level changed since I've started strength training?

    » *Be sure you're getting all the quality sleep that you need.*

5. Am I able to follow the exercise instructions well enough to feel like I'm doing them properly?

    » *It may be a good idea to look over the exercises on a no-exercise day to be sure you understand how to do them.*

NOTES

Inspiration for This Week

If you think lifting is dangerous, try being weak. Being weak is dangerous.

–BRET CONTRERAS, SPORTS SCIENTIST

chapter 6

Week 3

Again, we will be working out three days this week, and doing two sets of each exercise, with a minute in between sets. Be sure you are fatiguing the working muscles with the 12-repetition range by choosing the appropriate weight or resistance, whether at home or in the gym.

To increase the weight on machines, simply add another weight plate to the stack. Some machines have the option of increasing by 5 lb increments. This is a safe way to start.

For the home workouts, we will be working with body weight, dumbbells, and resistance bands. To increase resistance with dumbbells, choose a heavier dumbbell. For resistance bands, either choose a heavier band, or adjust your grasp to shorten the amount of band being used. Don't forget to have fun!

WEEK 3: HOME WORKOUT

Day of the Week: Choose three days for this week's workout, with a day of rest between workouts.

Approximate Workout Time: 35 minutes (including 5-minute warm-up and 10-minute cooldown)

Overview: Bodyweight, dumbbells, and bands. Three sets of 12 repetitions (both sides) with 1 minute rest between sets.

Reminder: Warm-up, page 22; Cooldown, pages 22 to 41

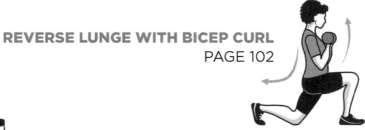

REVERSE LUNGE WITH BICEP CURL
PAGE 102

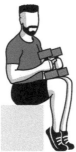

DUMBBELL CALF RAISES
PAGE 90

BENT-OVER ROW WITH RESISTANCE BANDS
PAGE 118

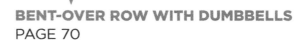

OR

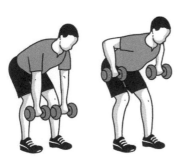

BENT-OVER ROW WITH DUMBBELLS
PAGE 70

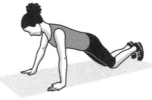

PUSH-UP FROM KNEES
PAGE 52

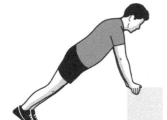

OR (more challenging)

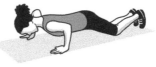

PUSH-UP FROM CHAIR
PAGE 54

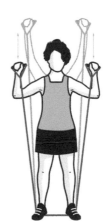

**STANDING OVERHEAD PRESS
WITH LIGHT RESISTANCE BAND**
PAGE 120

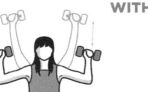

OR

**STANDING OR SEATED
OVERHEAD PRESS
WITH DUMBBELLS**
PAGE 78

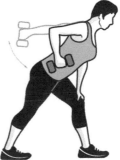

**SINGLE-ARM TRICEPS KICKBACK
WITH LIGHT DUMBBELL**
PAGE 80

WEEK 3: GYM WORKOUT

Day of the Week: Choose three days for this week's workout, with a day of rest between workouts.

Approximate Workout Time: 35 minutes (including 5-minute warm-up and 10-minute cooldown)

Overview: Dumbbells and machines. Three sets of 12 repetitions (both sides) with 1 minute rest between sets.

Reminder: Warm-up, page 22; Cooldown, pages 22 to 41

SQUATS WITH OVERHEAD PRESS
PAGE 104

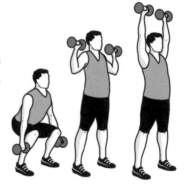

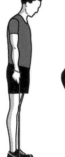
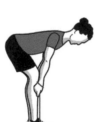

ROMANIAN DEADLIFT
PAGE 130

LAT PULL-DOWN MACHINE
PAGE 134

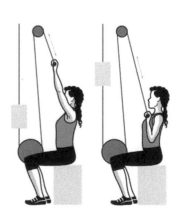

SEATED CABLE ROW ON MACHINE
PAGE 136

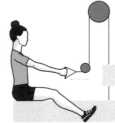

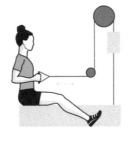

OR

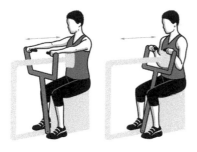

SEATED ROW ON FIXED MACHINE
PAGE 138

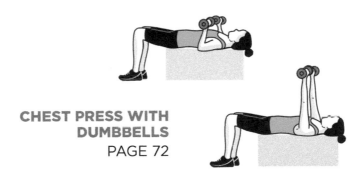

CHEST PRESS WITH DUMBBELLS
PAGE 72

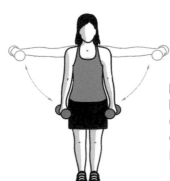

LATERAL SHOULDER RAISE WITH DUMBBELLS
(you may also do these seated on a stability ball or weight bench)
PAGE 76

SELF CHECK-IN WORKSHEET

1. Am I putting enough effort into each exercise, so that those last couple of repetitions are hard work?

   » *Let yourself be at least a little bit uncomfortable. It's not supposed to be easy.*

2. How do I feel just prior to working out as opposed to just after?

   » *We often say that no one ever said, "I wish I didn't do that workout!"*

3. Am I keeping a record of my workout weights?

   » *It is very motivational to see the numbers increase even a little.*

4. Do I find myself focusing too much on the scale?

   » *Remember that we are focusing on strength. I often tell my clients that if we focus on getting stronger, everything else will just naturally follow.*

5. Do I find myself more aware of my body? Do I feel like I'm aware of muscles I didn't know I had?

   » *One of the great things about strength training is that we become more aware of our bodies and how we move.*

Notes

Inspiration for This Week

You will not always be motivated. That's where discipline comes in.

–ALANA COLLINS

chapter 7

Week 4

We will be working out three days this week and increasing to three sets of each exercise, with 45 to 60 seconds of rest between sets. Be sure you are fatiguing the working muscles with the 12-repetition range. If you find three sets are too challenging this week, no problem. Continue with two sets this week and try for three sets next week.

Work out with more intensity this week. If using dumbbells, try increasing the weight. If using bands, try increasing the resistance by adjusting the amount of play you have with the band. Also attempt all the exercises *without* modifications. It's not supposed to be easy. Don't be afraid of having to work hard for those last couple of repetitions without losing form. Always maintain control of the weight and movement. If you find you're losing control, it's time to stop that set.

OK, it's week FOUR. We're halfway there. You're AMAZING!

WEEK 4: HOME WORKOUT

Day of the Week: Choose three days for this week's workout, with a day of rest between workouts.

Approximate Workout Time: 45 minutes (including 5-minute warm-up and 10-minute cooldown)

Overview: Bodyweight, dumbbells, and bands. Three sets of 12 repetitions (both sides) with 45 seconds of rest between sets.

Reminder: Warm-up, page 22; Cooldown, pages 22 to 41

SQUATS WITH OVERHEAD PRESS
PAGE 104

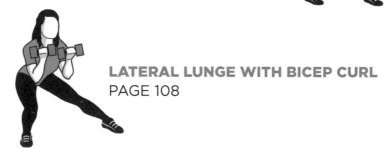

LATERAL LUNGE WITH BICEP CURL
PAGE 108

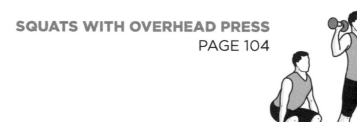

ROMANIAN DEADLIFT WITH RESISTANCE BANDS OR DUMBBELLS
PAGE 130

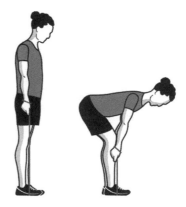

BENT-OVER ROW WITH DUMBBELLS OR RESISTANCE BAND
PAGE 70

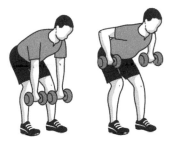

PUSH-UP FROM CHAIR
PAGE 54

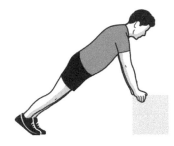

PULL-APARTS
PAGE 112

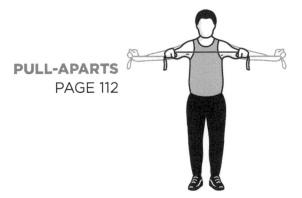

WEEK 4: GYM WORKOUT

Day of the Week: Choose three days for this week's workout, with a day of rest between workouts.

Approximate Workout Time: 45 minutes (including 5-minute warm-up and 10-minute cooldown)

Overview: Dumbbells and machines. Three sets of 12 repetitions (both sides) with 45 seconds of rest between sets.

Reminder: Warm-up, page 22; Cooldown, pages 22 to 41

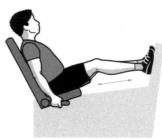

LEG PRESS MACHINE
PAGE 140

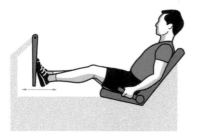

CALF RAISES ON LEG PRESS MACHINE
(be sure to increase the weight from week 1 superset [leg press/calf raise, leg press/calf raise])
PAGE 142

OR
(Non-machine alternative)

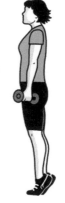 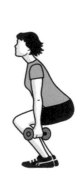

SQUAT TO CALF RAISE
PAGE 92

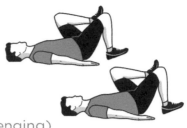

SINGLE-LEG GLUTE BRIDGE
PAGE 68

OR
(If single-leg is too challenging)

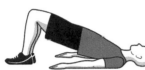

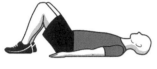

**GLUTE BRIDGE WITH
TWO FEET ON THE FLOOR**
PAGE 66

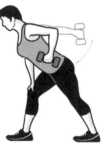

SINGLE-ARM TRICEPS KICKBACK
PAGE 80

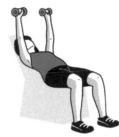

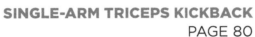

INCLINE CHEST PRESS
PAGE 74

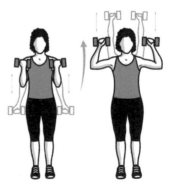

BICEP CURL TO SHOULDER PRESS
PAGE 84

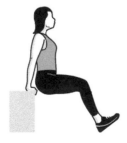

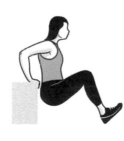

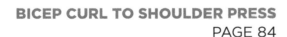

TRICEPS DIP ON BENCH
(try to extend legs in front
of you for more of a challenge)
PAGE 56

SELF CHECK-IN WORKSHEET

1. Do I notice how sleep, or lack thereof, affects my strength and endurance?

    » *Sleep has a significant impact on muscle recovery. If you don't get enough sleep, you're not going to feel rested in the morning, and your muscles will not recover properly.*

2. How has my strength training affected my appetite?

    » *Many people report that they are hungrier when they strength train, but the types of food they crave are generally healthier options.*

3. Am I finding myself researching (on social media, YouTube, etc.) more about strength training? Am I talking to my family and friends about strength training?

    » *The more you know, the more reasons you'll find to keep it up. I recommend Jeff Cavaliere (AthleanX.com) on YouTube for the best strength training advice.*

4. Do I find on days that I exercise, I crave more water?

    » *You know that growing muscles require lots of protein, but they need even more water.*

Notes

Inspiration for This Week

The more difficult the victory, the greater the happiness in winning.

-PELÉ

chapter

8

Week 5

This week we will complete three sets of 10 to 12 repetitions for each exercise, with about 45 seconds of rest between sets, whether exercising at home or in the gym. The lower rep range should enable you to increase the weight or resistance a little. If you cannot increase the weight, slow the motion down. I will talk more about that in week 6.

I invite you to look at the core (abdominal and lower back) exercises in chapter 3, to familiarize yourself with them. We *do* engage our core muscles while strength training, even while focusing on other muscle groups, but some of us feel the need to add core-specific exercises to our workouts. I suggest choosing one or two of the core exercises from chapter 3 and incorporating them into your strength training regime this week or doing them on alternate days.

Here we are in week FIVE. Give yourself a pat on the back. You deserve it!

WEEK 5: HOME WORKOUT

Day of the Week: Choose three days for this week's workout, with a day of rest between workouts.

Approximate Workout Time: 45 minutes (including 5-minute warm-up and 10-minute cooldown)

Overview: Bodyweight, dumbbells, and bands. Three sets of 10 to 12 repetitions (both sides) with 45 seconds of rest between sets. Increase the weight if you can. Include one set each of two core exercises (chapter 3) this week, whether on workout days or alternate days (see page 46).

Reminder: Warm-up, page 22; Cooldown, pages 22 to 41

LATERAL LUNGE WITH BICEP CURL
PAGE 108

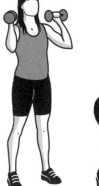 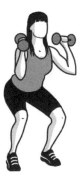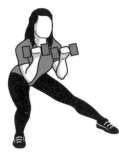

DUMBBELL SQUATS
PAGE 94

DUMBBELL CALF RAISES
PAGE 90

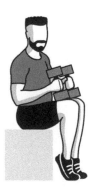

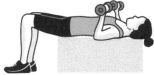

**CHEST PRESS
WITH DUMBBELLS**
PAGE 72

OR

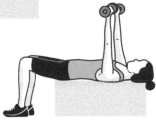

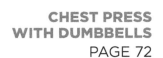

**PUSH-UPS FROM TOES
WITH REST AT THE BOTTOM**
PAGE 55

**STANDING OR SEATED OVERHEAD PRESS
WITH DUMBBELLS**
PAGE 78

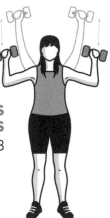

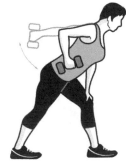

**SINGLE-ARM TRICEPS
KICKBACK WITH DUMBBELL
OR RESISTANCE BAND**
PAGE 80

WEEK 5: GYM WORKOUT

Day of the Week: Choose three days for this week's workout, with a day of rest between workouts.

Approximate Workout Time: 45 minutes (including 5-minute warm-up and 10-minute cooldown)

Overview: Dumbbells and machines. Three sets of 10 to 12 repetitions (both sides) with 45 seconds of rest between sets. Increase the weight if you can. Include one set each of two core exercises (chapter 3) this week, whether on workout days or alternate days (see page 46).

Reminder: Warm-up, page 22; Cooldown, pages 22 to 41

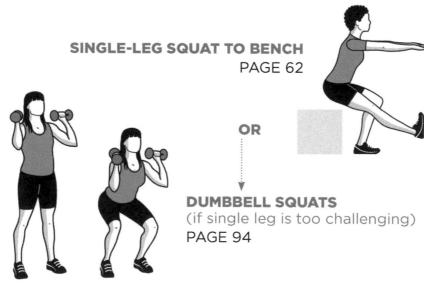

SINGLE-LEG SQUAT TO BENCH
PAGE 62

OR

DUMBBELL SQUATS
(if single leg is too challenging)
PAGE 94

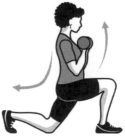

REVERSE LUNGE WITH BICEP CURL
PAGE 102

SINGLE-LEG DEADLIFT
PAGE 96

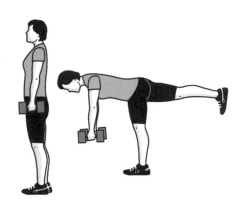

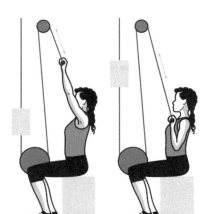

LAT PULL-DOWN MACHINE
PAGE 134

INCLINE CHEST PRESS ON BENCH
PAGE 74

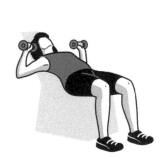

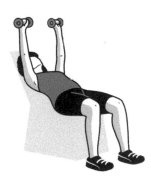

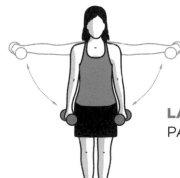

LATERAL SHOULDER RAISE WITH DUMBBELLS
PAGE 76

SELF CHECK-IN WORKSHEET

1. Did I exercise with as much intensity as I could have?

    » *If not, was it lack of energy? Or was I lacking motivation? It's important to get proper rest and nutrition so that we have the physical energy to exercise. Otherwise any excuse will do.*

2. Did I set and maintain high standards for myself with my nutrition this week?

    » *If not, was it because of a lack of worthy examples? If so, seek inspiration. What similar feats of accomplishment have inspired you in the past? What standards did those people set for themselves?*

3. Was I sure to carve out enough time in my day to exercise? Did I plan my day ahead so that I was sure to allow time to exercise?

    » *Using time efficiently is a skill that is acquired over time. It takes practice and discipline to learn how to use your time wisely, but if we want something bad enough, we will make time. It comes down to what is truly important to you.*

4. Was I able to regulate procrastination, distractions, and temptations in order to stay on track with sleep, nutrition, and exercise?

    » *For me, being successful with my strength training is about making my health and well-being a priority. There will be some trial and error at first, until you strike the right balance.*

Notes

Inspiration for This Week

If you are working on something exciting that you really care about, you don't have to be pushed. The vision pulls you.

-STEVE JOBS

Week 6

You have made it to week 6! I want to sincerely express just how proud I am of you. This week we will continue working within the 10 to 12 repetitions with a short rest: no more than 45 seconds between sets. At the risk of repeating myself, I want to remind you to choose a weight that *challenges* the muscles within that rep range. This is how we get stronger.

In this last week, we are focusing on the intensity of our workouts. It's a *fact* that building strength has more to do with intensity than simply going through the motions. We will now pay attention to something known as "time under tension," or TUT, which is commonly used in more advanced strength training.

How do we incorporate "time under tension"? Easy, just go slower. Focus on the muscles you're using and take your time.

WEEK 6: HOME WORKOUT

Day of the Week: Schedule three days for this week's workout, with a day of rest between workouts.

Approximate Workout Time: 45 minutes (including 5-minute warm-up and 10-minute cooldown)

Overview: Bodyweight, dumbbells, and bands. Three sets of 10 to 12 repetitions (both sides) with a maximum of 45 seconds of rest between sets. Increase the weight if you can. Focus on time under tension. Include one set each of two core exercises (chapter 3) this week, whether on workout days or alternate days (see page 46).

Reminder: Warm-up, page 22; Cooldown, pages 22 to 41

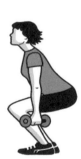
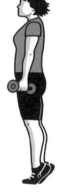

SQUAT TO CALF RAISE
PAGE 92

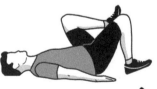

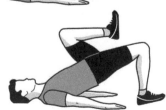

SINGLE-LEG GLUTE BRIDGE
PAGE 68

DO THE ONE THAT IS THE MOST
CHALLENGING FOR YOU

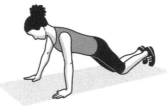

FLOOR PUSH-UP FROM KNEES
PAGE 52

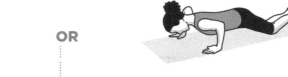

OR

**CHAIR PUSH-UP
WITH STRAIGHT LEGS**
PAGE 54

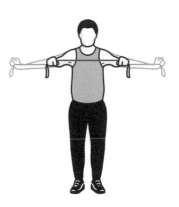

PULL-APARTS WITH RESISTANCE BAND
PAGE 112

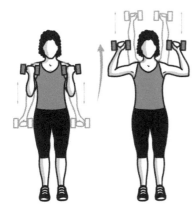

BICEP CURL TO SHOULDER PRESS
PAGE 84

**STANDING OVERHEAD TRICEPS EXTENSION
WITH EITHER A HEAVIER SINGLE DUMBBELL
OR ONE IN EACH HAND**
PAGE 82

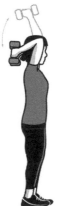

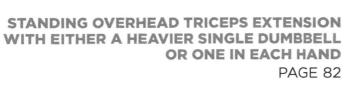

WEEK 6: GYM WORKOUT

Day of the Week: Choose three days for this week's workout, with a day of rest between workouts.

Approximate Workout Time: 45 minutes (including 5-minute warm-up and 10-minute cooldown)

Overview: Dumbbells and machines. Three sets of 10 to 12 repetitions (both sides) with 45 seconds of rest between sets. Increase the weight if you can. Focus on time under tension. Include one set each of two core exercises (chapter 3) this week, whether on workout days or alternate days (see page 46).

Reminder: Warm-up, page 22; Cooldown, pages 22 to 41

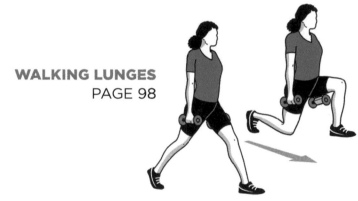

WALKING LUNGES
PAGE 98

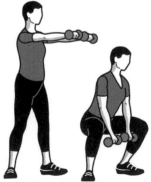

SUMO SQUATS WITH FRONT SHOULDER RAISE
PAGE 106

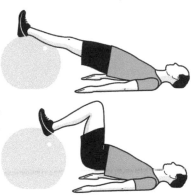

HAMSTRING ROLL-IN WITH STABILITY BALL
PAGE 128

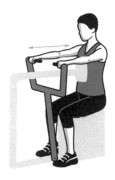 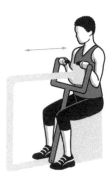

SEATED ROW (EITHER ON CABLE MACHINE OR FIXED MACHINE)
(be sure to increase the weight from week 3)
PAGE 138

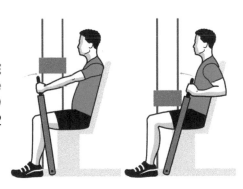

CHEST PRESS MACHINE
(be sure to increase the weight from week 1)
PAGE 132

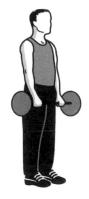 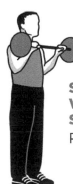

STANDING BICEP CURL WITH DUMBBELLS OR SMALL BARBELL
PAGE 86

SELF CHECK-IN WORKSHEET

1. What is the biggest lesson I learned about myself these past six weeks?

   » *Oftentimes, we learn the most important lessons about ourselves when we step outside of our comfort zones.*

2. Which seems more favorable to me: the pain of effort and discipline, or the pain of regret?

   » *I love the expression "I'd rather have a bunch of 'Oh wells' than a bunch of 'If onlys.'" In other words, go for it!*

3. Am I proud of my efforts?

   » *The payoff is always worthwhile when we follow through with something, especially if it is something new and unfamiliar. The most fulfilling reward is renewed confidence in ourselves.*

4. Am I truly ready to accept sustainable change in my life?

   » *No change will happen if we are not mentally prepared. We must be willing to let go of old habits that are keeping us stuck in old ways that no longer serve us.*

Notes

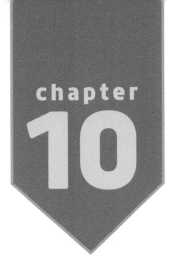

KEEP IT UP

I hope that you are feeling fabulous and reaping all the benefits of strength training. You may be sleeping better, eating better, feeling less pain in your body, and generally feeling more energetic and confident. You have a lot to be proud of.

It is important to now focus on *why* you want to maintain a strong, healthy body. The motivation may change over time, and some days you might not feel any motivation at all. That, my friends, is where discipline comes in.

WHAT'S NEXT?

You've reached the end of six weeks of strength training. Congratulations! However, this is not the end. Rather, it is the beginning of a whole new way of living.

Remember, your body *wants* to move. Your body wants to be strong. No matter your shape, size, age, or gender, if you love your body by giving it the opportunity to be strong and functional, the rewards will be invaluable.

I encourage you to go back to the beginning and start again, but this time, increase the weight and resistance. You may also do your favorite workouts for up to four weeks before switching to another.

Now that you've completed the foundation, feel free to use the exercises within this book to design your own programs, but be sure to include all of the necessary body parts. For strength training, we generally want to include at least two exercises for the legs and glutes, at least two for the back (pull), one or two for the chest (push), and an exercise for the shoulders or arms (biceps and triceps).

Always keep in mind that in order to get stronger you must lift more weight and gradually add more volume, making your muscles work harder than what they're used to. Listen to your body. It will tell you when to rest or to push a little harder.

SELF-STUDY FOR A STRONG LIFE

"No pain, no gain" is a popular mantra in the gym, although it can be misconstrued as a reason to overlook signs that your body needs a break. Some things to watch out for are persistent soreness or stiffness, and sharp, or persistent, nagging pain. If you're starting a new exercise, it's normal to be a little sore for up to 48 hours afterward. But if you're sore every time you do an exercise, that's when it's time to take notice. Other than the burning sensation of muscular fatigue, you shouldn't be feeling actual pain when you work out. If you have pain that persists even after you try to give that joint or muscle a rest, it's a good idea to get checked out by a physician.

Excessive fatigue can mean that you're overtraining. Give yourself an additional rest day, but again, if it persists you should check in with your physician.

Likewise, if you experience dizziness or fainting, be sure you are well-hydrated and not working out too hard. Exercising too hard can cause your blood pressure to drop or result in dehydration. This can leave you feeling lightheaded, dizzy, or faint. We don't want any of this.

BUILD A SUPPORT SYSTEM

It's my hope that you will be inspired to ask others to join you on this journey for a stronger body. There is someone just waiting for you to inspire them.

Seek out others who are on a similar path. Join a hiking group or invite a friend to go for a walk instead of sitting in a café. One of the great things about joining a gym is that those like-minded people are there for you.

Social media groups are also an awesome resource for inspiration. You'll find tons of support there, if that's something you enjoy. The point is to surround yourself with people who want you to succeed. Those people are your tribe.

ENJOY YOUR NEW SUPERPOWERS

I am often asked what my "secret" is, and without hesitation I answer, "Strength training!" I am positive I would not be the strong, capable woman I am today without it.

Just the other day I found myself in a situation where I had to climb over my seven-foot fence, clamber over my garden shed, and lower myself down using my upper body strength. I did it with such ease and felt like a giddy 12-year-old girl. I couldn't have done that had I not been so devoted to my strength training.

You may never find yourself in that situation but you *will* find that you are so much more capable of doing things that you thought you'd never be able to do again, and you will be able to continue doing the things you love for a long time to come.

Taking care of ourselves, especially as we age, is the *least* selfish thing we can do. Not only will we be able to keep up with children and grand-children, we will retain our independence for much longer, which are gifts to ourselves and the people we love.

WEBSITES

GirlsGoneStrong.com: Girls Gone Strong empowers women to be their strongest self. Get strength training tips, nutrition plans, and enroll in programs with top fitness trainers.

Greatist.com/fitness/resistance-band-exercises: Health and fitness news, tips, recipes, and exercises.

NerdFitness.com: A fitness website for nerds and average Joes. Helping you lose weight, get stronger, and live better.

NiaShanks.com: A no-nonsense approach to fitness and nutrition. Nia is a personal trainer dedicated to showing women how to build a better body by following a simple approach to nutrition and strength training.

YOUTUBE

Jeff Cavaliere, ATHLEAN-X
YouTube.com/channel/UCe0TLA0EsQbE-MjuHXevj2A
Jeff received his master's degree in physical therapy and bachelor of science in physio-neurobiology/pre-medicine from the University of Connecticut in Storrs, CT (one of the top five universities in the country in physical therapy and sports medicine).

James Linker, Shredded Sports Science
YouTube.com/channel/UCXrqErU_TjqiHAHJkzITAvg
James keeps the fitness industry honest with his lighthearted, yet science-based approach.

BOOKS

The Resistance Band Workout Book. **Ed McNeely and David Sandler. Burford Books.** More than 70 resistance band exercises, with step-by-step photos.

*Strength Band Training***, Second Edition. Phil Page and Todd S. Ellenbecker. Human Kinetics.** Shows you how to maximize strength, speed, and power in the gym, at home, or on the road with resistance bands.

*Strength Training Anatomy***, Third Edition. Frédéric Delavier. Human Kinetics.** In my opinion, this is the best anatomy book for those who would like to learn more about strength training.

Strength Training Nutrition 101: Build Muscle & Burn Fat Easily . . . A Healthy Way of Eating You Can Actually Maintain. **Marc McLean. CreateSpace.** A sensible, manageable nutrition guide that will help you get the most from your strength training program.

Younger Next Year: The Exercise Program. **Chris Crowley and Henry S. Lodge. Workman Publishing.** Based on the science that shows how we can turn back our biological clocks by a combination of aerobics and strength fitness, it's a guide that will show you how to live with vibrancy, strength, endurance, confidence.

CHAPTER 1

Dorfman, Steve. "FAU Study Highlights How Muscle Mass and Brain Health Are Connected." *The Palm Beach Post*. Updated August 28, 2018. PalmBeachPost.com/news/how-muscle-massand-brain-healthare-connected/Jq9JoMypTxxcL2sw9n0dEP.

Harvard Medical School. "Strength Training Builds More Than Muscles." *Harvard Health Publishing* (blog). Accessed January 7, 2020. Health.Harvard.edu/staying-healthy/strength-training-builds-more-than-muscles.

Liu-Ambrose, Teresa. "How Exercise Can Boost Brain Power." *UBC News* (blog). February 6, 2014. News.UBC.ca/2014/02/06/how-exercise-can-boost-brain-power.

University of Eastern Finland. "Greater Muscle Strength, Better Cognitive Function for Older People." *ScienceDaily*. June 26, 2017. ScienceDaily.com/releases/2017/06/170626093546.htm.

Webber, Sandra C, Michelle M. Porter, and Verena H. Menec. "Mobility in Older Adults: A Comprehensive Framework." *The Gerontologist*, Volume 50, Issue 4. (August 2010): 443–450. Academic.OUP.com/gerontologist/article/50/4/443/743504.

CHAPTER 2

American Heart Association. "Prescription Omega-3 Medications Work for High Triglycerides." *American Heart Association News*. August 19, 2019. Heart.org/en/news/2019/08/19/prescription-omega3-medications-work-for-high-triglycerides-advisory-says.

CHAPTER 4

Larson, Christian D. "Believe in yourself and all that you are. Know that there is something inside you that is greater than any obstacle." Passiton.com. Accessed January 23, 2020. PassItOn.com/inspirational-quotes/6545-believe-in-yourself-and-all-that-you-are-know.

Wattpad. "10 Facts about Biology." WattPad.com/520446760-1-000-facts-about-everything-10-facts-about.

CHAPTER 5

Braathe, Robert. "Gratitude and attitude are not challenges; they are choices." En.WikiQuote.org/wiki/Gratitude.

CHAPTER 6

Contreras, Bret. Twitter post. April 7, 2014, Twitter.com/bretcontreras/status/453240488967958530?lang=en.

CHAPTER 8

Pele. "The more difficult the victory, the greater the happiness in winning." Google.com/books/edition/The_More_Difficult_the_Victory_the_Great/WvMvxwEACAAJ?hl=en.

CHAPTER 9

Jobs, Steve. "If you are working on something exciting that you really care about, you don't have to be pushed. The vision pulls you." Google.com/books/edition/Don_t_Quote_Me/Sq3YDQAAQBAJ?hl=en&gbpv=0.

INDEX

ACKNOWLEDGMENTS

I would like to thank all of my clients who have entrusted me with their fitness and, at the same time, taught me so much. They help me to be a better trainer and a better person, every day.

ABOUT THE AUTHOR

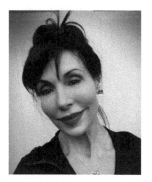 Alana Collins has been working as a Certified Fitness Coach in Victoria, British Columbia, since 2012. She works primarily with middle-aged and older women and men.

As a former figure skater, Alana found she could no longer compete with the girls with naturally strong legs as she approached her late-teen years. Determined to build strength, she joined a gym where she was often the only "girl" in the place. The gym has been a significant part of her life ever since.

Currently, Alana loves to help others be the best version of themselves by teaching them how to be strong. She is a proponent of strength training for *life*, rather than the quick-fix gimmicks. Her philosophy is to focus on strength rather than the scale, and the rest will fall into place.

Alana gave birth to her youngest child just days away from her 45th birthday and made a silent promise to him to stay strong for as long as she could.

For more information about Alana, visit her website AlanaCollinsFitness Coach.com.

Printed in the USA
CPSIA information can be obtained
at www.ICGtesting.com
LVHW081656301123
764704LV00004B/43

9 781646 116126